BREAK FREE FROM HEART ATTACK FEAR

THE SURVIVOR'S GUIDE TO EMBRACE YOUR TRUTH, REGAIN CONFIDENCE & RESTORE CONTROL

LISA STEELE GEORGE

Copyright © Lisa Steele George 2020

All rights reserved. No part of this book may be reproduced in any form without permission in writing from the author. Reviewers may quote brief passages in reviews.

Published 2020

DISCLAIMER

No part of this publication may be reproduced or transmitted in any form or by any means, mechanical or electronic, including photocopying or recording, or by any information storage and retrieval system, or transmitted by email without permission in writing from the author.

Neither the author nor the publisher assumes any responsibility for errors, omissions, or contrary interpretations of the subject matter herein. Any perceived slight of any individual or organization is purely unintentional.

All the names and identifying information in client stories have been changed. Stories shared about the author's experiences are detailed from her memories and her perspective only. Any resemblance in this book to real persons living or dead is purely coincidental apart from the author's own stories that are true to her.

This book contains discussions about health issues and medical problems. By reading this book, you acknowledge that the author is not a licensed psychologist, doctor, or other health care professional and the opinions in this book do not replace the care of psychologists, doctors, or other healthcare professionals. If you have questions about a medical problem, please refer to your doctor, psychologist, or other healthcare professional. The author's opinions in this book are in no way to be construed as or substituted for diagnosis, medical advice, psychological counseling, or any other type of therapy or cure. The author cannot guarantee the outcome of the coaching efforts and/ or recommendations in this book and her comments about the outcome are expressions of her opinion only. Also, please be advised that the author cannot be held responsible for the medical decisions that you make as a result of reading this book. Please consult your physician or healthcare provider before making any changes in your health habits or diet.

Brand and product names are trademarks or registered trademarks of their respective owners.

Contributing Authors: Courtney Steele George, Registered Dietitian, MPH Nutrition, UNC Chapel Hill; and Dalton Robert George, Ph.D., Applied Ethics & Policy of Biotechnology, NC State

Cover design by: Jennifer Stimson

Editor: Natasa Smirnov

Author's Photos: Jessica Stasik JLBoone Photography

My Heart is Free logo design by Allison McDonald Allspire Designs

CONTENTS

Foreword	xi
1. A Heart in Crisis	1
2. Pumphead	15
3. How to Read This Book	31
4. Step 1 – Understanding Heart Dis-Ease and the Shame Game	45
5. Step 2 – Light Science: Knowledge Is Power	61
6. Step 3 – Taking Inventory: Your Truth	79
7. Step 4 — Stages of Grief	93
8. Step 5 — Pillar People, Support Network & Get Organized	111
9. Step 6 — Unpack Your Crap	127
10. Step 7 – Recalibrate	139
11. Step 8 – Heart Connections	153
12. Step 9 – Post-Traumatic Growth	165
13. Step 10 – A Year of Gentleness	179
14. May Your Heart Soar	203
Appendix: Healthy Heart Nutrition	209
Acknowledgments	219
About the Author	221
About Difference Press	223
Other Books by Difference Press	225
Thank You	227

ADVANCE PRAISE

"I am so impressed, moved and uplifted! The candor of George's narrative is instantly relatable, and the paths she carves to help herself and others find truth in the 'Heart Healing Process' are applicable to anyone facing uncertainty following critical illness. This book, like the heart itself, is a roadmap showing where the highways of heart science intersect with new self-actualizing behaviors; how to expertly navigate your Truth like in the face of a surprise construction zone; and when to take heed of stop signs telling you to pause, re-assess your goals and the environment around you, and proceed with confidence towards a new destination that awaits you....this work of art that has emerged from (her) mind and heart!"

— Dr. Vasiliki Nataly Rahimzadeh, PhD Postdoctoral Fellow, Stanford Center for Biomedical Ethics, Stanford University

"Very enjoyable book! Those who have had heart attacks will be able to relate at a deep level to everything she writes about and those who haven't are in for an empowering and inspiring read. Lisa's personal stories really help you feel and understand her experience in having a heart attack. That street cred makes her advice meaningful and relevant."

— Brian Granader, Owner of Red Lotus Yoga Studio, Rochester Hills, Michigan

"I really enjoyed reading this! *Break from Heart Attack Fear* is a book that answers many important questions for individuals that have either survived a heart attack or for individuals who care for a loved one recovering from a heart attack. Lisa covers the nutrition, exercise, and mental wellbeing. She explores and answers many questions that truly matter. Her approach to such a challenging topic is practical, solid, and empowering. Lisa's story provides readers with absorbing and valuable insight into heart dis-ease, and being able to reach one's full potential."

— Josephine R. Cervantes, MA, LPC, NCC, Clinical Psychology Doctoral Candidate

*This book is dedicated to my Sun-Son Dalton Robert
and my Soul-Sole Spirit daughter Courtney Steele.
I'm in awe of the gifts you share with the world,
your dedication to being change agents for this planet
and humbled by the way you hold space for me.
You have my deep love, devotion and gratitude always.
Thank you for showing me how to embrace my Truth.*

FOREWORD

In my sixty-two years, I have mothered five children, studied business, neuroscience, health, nutrition, Brainspotting, and Yoga. I've traveled the globe to experience many diverse cultures, as well as offer services to those in need in third world countries. I am the founder of Whole Life Healing Centers, a non-profit organization focused on providing services for victims of domestic violence, sex trafficking, and veterans suffering from PTSD. Above all else, loving others has always been my passion and purpose in life!

In 2011, one of my younger brothers passed away from a heart attack. My world spun and crashed around me, like it has for many of you who are about to embark upon reading this heart-felt, informative and captivating book. Had I found this book back then, and better understood all the content of this book, I might be able to tell you that my own health wasn't affected, and that things turned out differently for me than they did. But they did not. I suffered from a stroke just eight months after my brother died. My body was simply not able to handle the emotional pain from his heart event and overwhelming life stressors I was forced to experience. Like many of you, I found myself in a new and different life-threatening situation from both my brother's heart attack death and then the stroke. While much of the ensuing months were filled with confusion and unclear thoughts, one thought was very clear: I needed to get well, I needed to heal. It was as if the Neuroscience Life Coaching studies from my past were meant just for this time, my now!

While in the hospital, as many of you, including Lisa, also experienced, a disbelief and an unwillingness to accept the reality of what was happening is true of my own story. Yet, somehow in the midst of laying in the hospital, I heard the whisper of God from deep within: "Study. Use your brain. Visualize. Create new connections in your brain". While I knew this was possible, at the time, my thoughts were not very cohesive. But I listened to that whisper the best I could, given my condition. Just like Lisa, who started the beginning of her book through her journaling while in the hospital post heart attack, I began to study right there in my hospital bed, post stroke, to stimulate my brain. Truth be told, I haven't stopped studying since!

My brain did get better, just like a heart can, and even though I am not the same person I was before the stroke, I survived and am here to share the story and dedicate my life to the service and helping others, very similar to Lisa's journey. We both share the same, strong philosophies that recovery is required for full healing, that our body wants the best health for us and that these types of crisis events bring us to a new 'me/you', a wonderful journey.

I was able to continue my career, studying with Dr. Daniel Amen at the Institute of Integrative Nutrition (IIN) with further studies at the Centre for Applied Neuroscience (CAN). I traveled to India to study yoga with a Catholic Priest and upon my return, my coaching practice grew, grandchildren were added, and my life became full once again.

Then in July of 2019, I had trouble breathing. I thought it was just my asthma and treated it as such, passing it off with excuses, just as Lisa talks about so very well in her work. One night, I couldn't carry myself and my little 8 lb. dog up the stairs. Instead, I had to sit on my bum and go up the stairs backwards, one step at a time. The next day, I called my doctor. He wanted to see me right away, but I told him I'd come the next day because I had a full load of clients for work that day. I will not take anything away from the brilliance in this book, but if you are reading this and resonating with the denial I was in, I highly suggest you ingest every word Lisa shares with you. While I did not have a heart attack, I had a virus that 'attacked' my heart and put me in congestive heart failure. How could this have happened to me, again? Me, the Coach training other Coaches. The Intuitive Eating Coach. The Neuroscience Coach. The well-established yoga instructor. Once again, I found myself flabbergasted at what was happening to me. The whirlwind of tests. The grim predictions of my future. Had there been a book like this book, "Break Free from Heart Attack Fear" that I had read, I would have internalized its content and taken its wisdom to heart. I would have done things differently, both times around, that would have yielded better choices and outcomes. This second crisis for me, though, didn't bring denial with it. Instead, it was acceptance. I worked with my body and the belief that I could and would get well - no matter what anyone told me. And get well I did – to *everyone*'s surprise, except my holistic doctor, Dr. David Brownstein, who literally helped to save my life!

Then Lisa Steele George walks into my life. A mutual friend recommended she attend my Whole Life Healing Wellness coaching program. We spoke a few months after the heart attack that had changed her life. She expressed that she needed deep self-development work right now. I could see right away that she was one of those rare people who come into your life, never leaving it the same because she touches it with something extra special and unique. Lisa joined my coaching course. Her determination and tenacity to heal was striking. We met for one weekend a month for 6 months with a lot of homework in between. What I respect most is Lisa's willingness to *be* herself. She allowed not only for her body to heal and receive whatever she needed, while she also worked very diligently on her inner emotional healing and wounds. It was a beautiful process to watch her bloom over those six months.

The best part is she didn't stop there. Lisa told me the first time we met that she was going to write a book. And here we are, with me writing a foreword for that very book. What comes next, under this beautiful cover, are words and processes that draw you into her experience. She helps you connect to the emotional pieces of the experience of a heart attack, but she doesn't leave you there. She provides brilliant advice for your whole-body health and encourages you to make the choices that will support you. Her words will touch your soul and the wisdom that lies herein has the ability to create change for you, the reader.

Last, but not least, for you Lisa, I wish you continued success on this beautiful journey of life. May your heart always be whole, and your life full. I have no doubt that many will be helped by your book and will seek your support as you gently guide them to discover their own healing path. You are truly an inspiration!

— Bethany Perry, CAN, IAHC, AAEC, ERYT Founder & CEO of Whole Life Healing Centers & Whole Life Healing Coaching Collective Intuitive Neuroscience Life Coach Certified Brainspotting Practitioner

1

A HEART IN CRISIS

"It's that heart of gold and stardust soul that makes you beautiful."

— R. M. BRODERICK

"Vampire Nurse" was her nickname. She strolled into our rooms by the hour, poking painful needles into our tender skin. "I'm taking your blood," she'd mutter out of her thick, red-lipstick-caked lips, "for the doctors, to measure your troponin levels." Every single time she returned to the room she would mutter this from a deep guttural level. Not a stitch of tenderness was invoked, not even the slightest intimation of compassion from her stone-colored eyes. For the next twelve hours, this torture went on, every hour on the hour. Her overbleached blonde hair swooped across her face in long layers against her pale, colorless cheeks. Her hair was lopsided. You knew it was a wig. Poke, poke, poke on the tender, thin-skinned tops of my hands, all over my arms, and sometimes my legs. *What is going on? How did I get here? What's happening?*

This creature just would not leave me alone. *Where was I? What is troponin?*

I woke up several times, in and out of long, dazed stupors. I was lying in a hospital bed, wrapped in a blood-stained hospital gown, feeling exhausted beyond any belief. *How did I get here?* It felt like there was a boulder weighing down my whole body because it was so tiring to even move a limb. My eyes would open and close, trying to bring on restful sleep while remaining conscious about what was going on around me. *Oh yeah,* I suddenly remembered. A doctor came in at some point during my fog. I'll never forget the words I heard floating in the air over to me: "You had a heart attack." *Was he talking to me? Or am I dreaming?* That's impossible.

Those are words that no one ever wants to hear. You physically hear them, the words travel into your ears, to your brain, but they don't register. The words don't stick in your brain, so you fall back to sleep. "What? Are you sure? Are you sure?" I repeated to him.

"Yes, most definitely," he answered. "We have your troponin levels back. It is a test that measures the proteins in your blood, which are released when the heart muscle has been damaged, occurring with a heart attack." I had never heard of this word, "troponin." *How do you say it? Trop-On-In? How will I even remember this?* I fell back to sleep.

A nurse explained to me that when someone has a heart attack or experiences any type of injury to the muscles of the heart, troponin levels quickly rise. Doctors measure troponin levels in the blood within hours of symptoms emerging in order to screen for life-threatening problems like a myocardial infarction (another word for heart attack). For some people who may have suffered a cardiac arrest with myocarditis (inflammation and damage of the heart muscle), medical attention can be received right away as a result of the troponin measurements, which can be life-saving.

I was in shock. I had only ever been in the hospital for delivery of my two babies. I had been in this hospital overnight already, since 2 p.m. the day before, Monday, October 28, 2019. Vampire Nurse was nowhere to be seen anymore. She had gotten all the blood from me that she needed. Thank God for that relief. The bruises all over my body were so tender and sensitive that it made getting comfortable impossible. Other medical professionals, though, streamed in and out of my room for the first twenty-four hours to poke more, ask questions, listen to my heart, and educate me about this so-called heart attack I had suffered. I tried to absorb as much as I could, but comprehension just was not possible. I needed help. It was time to call in the reinforcements: my kids. So, I did.

MOBILIZED RESCUE

I phoned both of my kids. My sun-son Dalton Robert was in Raleigh, completing his Ph.D. at North Carolina State in the field of Applied Ethics in Policy of Biotechnology. My sole-soul daughter Courtney Steele was near Raleigh at the University of North Carolina, Chapel Hill. She was working on completing her two master's degrees, one in Nutrition and the other in Public Health. It was really early in the morning, so I hoped I wouldn't be waking them up. They both answered sounding somewhat groggy, my son especially. He told me straight away that he had a horrid night of sleeping, tossing, and turning. They both said, right off, "Why are you calling so early? Why are you even up?"

I started with normal chitchat, not wanting to startle them right off the bat. I remember telling them both a quick version of what happened, with the goal of making it not sound too bad. In other words, sugarcoating things, a habit I've had my whole life. The people dearest to me know all too well that I have this habit, but how does one actually sugarcoat a conversation when it comes to heart attacks? I don't really remember. I just know that I didn't want to startle or shock them, so I gave a light version of the situation from the "protective mom" side that was in full throttle. "I had an issue with my heart," I told them. "But it's all going to be fine."

"Mom, are you saying you had a heart attack; that you are in the hospital? What did the doctor actually call it, Mom?" Dalton asked.

"Um, something like a myo-card fraction," I replied

"OK, Mom. That's a heart attack. Myocardial infarction is a heart attack, Mom. You had a heart attack." A dead silence followed for a short while. "Let me call you back," he finally said.

The next call I got from him was an hour later. This time on his cell phone speaker in his car. Within that hour, my sun-son had packed his critical stuff, driven to Carrboro to pick up his soul-sole sister, and fully mobilized a trip up north to Michigan to be with me.

Wow, I thought, *this must be serious.* I was a fifty-six-year-old woman, lying in a hospital bed, recovering from what was called a "myocardial infarction (MI)," waiting for my two adult kids to come to be with me. *How the hell did this happen?* But here come my angels to the rescue!

I lay in my bed for mere hours, hooked up to all sorts of IVs, testing gadgets, and cuffs, dazed and trying to remember the details. Everything still seemed fuzzy. I ached all over. I couldn't get comfortable with all the equipment and needles attached to me and those constant beeps assuring everyone that my heart was still beating. The other sounds in the room were from machines I had never seen, but were still reminders that I was indeed in a hospital room. I started thinking of the name the doctor used for my diagnosis. I still could not say the words heart attack, or the other one that was hard to pronounce: myocardial infarction. *Which one did I have? Were they the same? Was one worse than the other?* I was clearly in shock because I kept waiting for a doctor to come in and tell me that they had given me the wrong information, with the wrong results that were meant for someone else. I was convinced that I really had walking pneumonia or some other illness. I decided to get some rest. After all, my kids will sort it out when they get here, I reassured myself. They are so smart with the science. They have always been the science ones. They will be able to get to the bottom of this phony craziness.

As time passed and hours on the clock kept ticking by, I realized I was involuntarily embarking on a new journey that was starting in this hospital. I always use the words "journey" or "adventure" to describe unfolding experiences in my life. My all-time favorite word, though – that my kids can attest to – is "process." From the time the kids were little, I would often say to them, "Be patient, sweetheart. It's a process." Or "Remain mindful and observe how the process unfolds." The best one yet was, "Life is a process! Enjoy it!" It's still a joke between us. Now, when I hear them using the word *process* to describe an experience, I chuckle inside.

There I was, enduring a lot of *processes* in the midst of my hospital adventure while on a new *journey*. *Oh, what joy,* I thought sarcastically. I was told that I would be there for a while, as tests and multiple procedures needed to be completed. There also had to be time enough to sort out what medications were required, what combination of meds, their schedule, and any reactions I might have to them. The most critical factor for being there was for observation, to ensure another heart attack wasn't on the horizon.

I eventually resigned myself to the idea that I was not going home anytime soon. This was when the fear and shock started to set in for me. It started to feel all too real now. I tried to keep my chin up, facing the situation like an explorer of new lands, asking questions of the medical staff, being curious enough but not annoying, laughing at their jokes and even allowing the resident doctors to come in and use me as their guinea pig. The same response occurred every time a new person came into my room. They would look at me and say, "Wow, you're too young to have had a heart attack!" or "You're the youngest heart attack patient I've ever had!" being all excited about my condition. This left me feeling even more conflicted.

FEAR AND SHOCK

As the fear continued to bubble up, I realized that this was a foreign land, a place I had never been before, with an unknown culture. I wondered if I had the courage to face it. *Where did all my yoga practice mindfulness go? Where was that strength?* For ten years I had been practicing and teaching yoga on and off. I should have had the tools and the skills to wade through these waters with confidence, but for whatever reason, they just were not rising up within me. I was too overwhelmed with so many emotions; I couldn't muster anything up that was in the least bit yoga-ish.

Instead, fear, shock, and sadness were creeping in by the hour and I was forced, by circumstance, to connect with the unknown hospital-land. I was forced to go beneath the surface of the sugarcoated rendition I had created of my situation and face the Truth, with a capital

"T" of this Trauma, also with a capital "T." Would I have an earthshaking revelation that would rescue me from the gates of this hell? Would I suddenly find something deep inside me that would bring me immediate reprieve? Would I realize that yes, indeed, all of life is filled with impermanence and this is just another example, so accept it? No, nothing like this was happening. Instead, I had monkey-mind, with one thought constantly leaping to yet another. Questions remained unanswered and all I could do was lay in my bed, listening to the sounds from the hospital hallway.

There is a ton of shock, denial, and twinges of embarrassment when a person suffers a heart attack. Maybe this is how you or your loved one felt. You lie there in your hospital bed and gown wondering how this ever could have happened. Where did you lose it enough to fall apart, causing a heart attack? You hear what the doctors are telling you but can't really comprehend it. Thoughts and feelings reside deeply and bubble up more as the reality of the situation sets in. Most everyone feels this way, no matter their walk of life, age, or gender. The most common reaction to a heart attack or heart event is denial. It is a natural reaction and a natural way to protect yourself. You are faced with so much pain all at once, you need to hide from it for a while to survive it all.

Look at me, a clear-cut example of being in denial. I continued waiting for the doctor to come in and say that they had it all wrong, that they had given me the wrong information, and that I was not a heart attack victim. I waited for this apology, expecting it to come at any moment. This is not uncommon. Almost every heart attack victim I've spoken to or read about has the same reaction. I had to ask myself, what was my heart telling me? The answer was, it was telling me that I had a heart attack, while my head told a different story. This went on for hours, until I finally realized that everyone in a room in this hall had suffered from a heart event. I was a resident of the cardiac wing. *Bam!* My world was blown apart.

All you want to do at a time like this is hide under your blankets, one of my go-to moves in times of high stress. Or, if it were possible, turn the clock back to make it all disappear, and be transported back to your old life where you felt in control, knew what was happening and, most importantly, had confidence in your body. You want to wake up the next morning in your own bed, at home, and discover that the heart attack was just a bad dream. But soon enough, you realize that indeed it did happen, and the nightmare left you shell-shocked. As part of the aftermath, you suffer from actual heartbreak, not the kind experienced from romantic relationships, but one that is much more literal.

TSUNAMI OF EMOTIONS

There is a tsunami of emotions running through your mind following a heart attack. This is common and you are not alone. Physically, you are going through so many changes. Hormones are fired up. Chemicals are rushing to your brain in your body's defense, as a result of the attack. Chemicals are reacting with new ones forming and ravaging through your body. Medications are being administered via IVs as well as from pills. A lot is going on and coming at you right now, internally and externally.

Because of all of this, it is not uncommon to feel confusion and have some cognitive challenges following a heart event or heart surgeries. You may have been rushed into surgery for a coronary artery bypass grafting, immediately following an ambulance ride. An emergency valve replacement might have taken place, or a surgical procedure to correct irregular heart rhythms, such as atrial fibrillation or ventricular tachycardia. Going from an ambulance gurney to being rushed to have bypass surgery or other surgeries is massively overwhelming, both to you and your loved ones. You have shock to deal with, alongside the shock your loved ones are facing. The level of shock is almost incomprehensible. Regardless of the exact situation, you are a victim, flooded with a kaleidoscope of emotions like anxiety, fear, hopelessness, shock, and denial. This is a direct result of the event you've suffered, one that has caused mega chaos in your world. You are suffering from trauma, which is quickly becoming part of your story.

There are defining moments in life that change you forever. Sometimes you know when they are happening, at the precise moment they unravel in front of your eyes, and this is one of those life-changing moments. It will not be until after you have had time to reel back, come down, to process and reflect upon it, that you realize the magnitude of its power. I knew this to be the case when the medics came barreling through my front door the day before, finding me on my white chez lounger being licked incessantly by my two dogs, yet not able to move a muscle. I looked up into their faces thinking, *WTF just happened?*

While you lay there in your hospital gown, you begin to think about all sorts of things and start wondering, like I did – maybe your load was simply too much to bear? Maybe, when your boss gave you thirty days to find another job the week prior, you experienced more stress cortisol raging through your body than you could handle. Perhaps a recent lack of self-care tipped the scales out of your favor. Or, did genetics finally catch up with you? Better yet, did you have symptoms for a while, including being exhausted, but pushed them off? It's exhausting just thinking about the possible reasons.

Whatever the case may be, these moments culminated into an experience that changed your life story forever and you are now beholden to it. Maybe, with time, it will turn itself into an awakening. Of course, you don't know that right now, while in the hospital. You don't know if you will find the courage to accept the meaning behind this crisis. Will you get your life back? Will you embrace the power to heal and live an abundant life? Yes, you will and you can. How do I know this? Because I was able to and you are deserving of this and very special.

I was so tired and continued resting, focusing my attention on my kids' arriving by the end of the day. My mind was spinning while I felt like a failure, a let-down, and so damaged physically and emotionally. I had some moments of clarity when I remembered some passages I read earlier that week written by Mother Teresa of Calcutta. Repeating it in my head, I realized a much deeper meaning was instilled in me and once again, the swirl of emotions started up again:

"Always have a cheerful smile.... Don't only give your care, but give your heart as well.... A clean heart is a free heart. A free heart can love…"

What happened to my clean heart? It's broken into pieces now and feels so far from being free. Will I have a clean heart once again, free from blockages, emotional and physical? Will I be healthy again, with lots left to give? Maybe this was a new start for me, a clean slate – a phrase a childhood friend of mine often said in times of stress. He'd say offering up a clean slate was a way of starting over in response to conflict or disagreement. It was a common practice in his family. *Is this my clean slate to start over again?* I wondered. My Birdland neighborhood friend also used to say, "I love you, Lisa. You have a golden heart." My heart didn't feel so golden at this time. It felt more like a wadded-up scrunch of tin foil. He was really telling me that my heart was kind and generous, since gold is something to be valued. I found comfort in remembering his words of long ago while lying in my hospital bed. Maybe he was right and this was a clean slate for me, with a lot left to do, to accomplish, new people to love, and fun life experiences to have. Maybe I did have value left even though everything had changed in a heartbeat.

There are so many feelings and reflections for heart attack survivors to have. One minute you can be on the brink of an existential crisis and in another, notice optimism creeping back in. This dynamic comes and goes. But the whole time, I felt deep within my heart that I would not only survive, but eventually I would thrive. Why? Because I decided that I would not give up, not as long as heartbeats vibrated through my chest. Not as long as my life force radiated through my heart in parallel with my breath. Not as long as my spirit restored my heart and filled it with continued hope and healing. Yes, change is taking place, but I will embrace it and continue to make shifts that are necessary for my well-being. I had decided that my life was not over. It was just a new beginning with a clean slate and a clean heart of gold – or soon to be literally cleaned. Once my kids got there to help me get my ducks in a row and organized, I was on my way to an abundant life.

WHY ME? WHY YOU?

Up until a heart attack, it felt like things like this happened to other people, but not to me or you because we were so blessed and lucky. We don't feel that way so much now.

But aren't we? Aren't we blessed to be recovering in a hospital? Aren't we still lucky because we are alive?

You then may ask, why now? Will I lose everything I've worked so hard for, in less than a week, from a heart attack I *wasn't* supposed to have? You may be feeling like you had such a bright future, but are now devastated by a questionable future. You may feel that you were taking care of yourself, you always played by the rules you were taught, and that this is just not fair. What are you supposed to do now with the stress, worry, and concerns that you are suddenly saddled with due to this unexpected nightmare?

Adversity will force you to face this trial, but you get to decide how to face it: either with courage and faith, or with fear and anxiety. It is your choice. You can work through this in order to land in a much better place when you get to the other side. This trial is taking you on a journey, a journey with a purpose. It is up to you to be patient enough that you can discover that purpose. It is up to you to endure this struggle with faith that this heart attack will bring you to a much better place. It is not meant to defeat you. There will be tiny miracles happening every day that will sustain you and move you in a better direction. You can choose to be open to these tiny miracles that will work on your behalf and help you to not only survive, but thrive. You do not need to dwell upon the negativity nor allow it to poison your whole being.

In this book, I will share with you how I have learned to achieve an abundant life after enduring my recovery, healing, and the first full year after my heart attack. Putting back order, fun, love, and health has been accomplished with confidence. In the following pages, I'm going to show you how to accomplish this through recovery and healing. It is not going to be easy, but having recurrent heart attacks is not an option, nor is staying on your couch for the rest of your life or isolating from the world out of fear. You can learn to push fear and worry away, and create a life filled with confidence and passion.

All victims are different and so were our heart events. But everyone comes to the table with one common denominator: being a survivor. What I do is guide survivors through the "Heart Healing Process (HHP)" to help move lives forward with confidence and excitement. You will stretch beyond the prison of your own beliefs and limitations, start living again, and doing the things you enjoy. While moving through this book, you will actually be making a transition to a transformed life, one that will better serve the new you and those you love. A clean slate. A new beginning.

2

PUMPHEAD

"There is no passion to be found in settling for a life that is less than the one you are capable of living."

— NELSON MANDELA

"They had to stop my heart you know. My breastbone was cut and divided in half, too. I was dead for a while. I don't feel like me anymore. Who am I? Why did this have to happen?" The guy from the next room told me. He'd had emergency bypass surgery. As a result, he was suffering from major depression and other kinds of moods that were new to him. We talked in the hall and I'll never forget how he described his experience, referring to it as his "first death." He believed the surgery left him with a mild case of an identity crisis.

His face looked so tired, many years beyond his actual age. I was shocked at hearing this and felt so sorry for him. He looked at me with sincere wonder and said, "Why are you here? You sick or something?" My head went down, and I quietly told him that I had something going on with my heart that needed checking out. I didn't tell him that I had a heart attack. I still couldn't say it. Admitting it was still an impossible act. The words simply would not roll off my tongue and out my mouth, even when I tried.

I was amazed that this guy could even walk a few steps, let alone share his event with me. This is what it's called in the heart attack world, an "event". Cardiovascular events refer to any type of interruption of the blood flow to the heart that ends up as an injury to the heart. An event can refer to a sudden cardiac arrest, where a person's heart stops pumping blood around the body. An event can also refer to other cardiovascular situations like acute coronary syndrome. I soon realized that I had to become familiar with many new words and definitions when living in Cardiac-ville.

It's of utmost importance for every victim to fully understand what happened to them, the underlying causes, diagnosis and condition(s) that they have to manage going forward. All too often, victims leave the hospital without knowing or really understanding what caused their event. They have some idea, but for ease and comfort, they simply leave it to having a heart attack. Unless underlying details are understood in full and given proper attention, healing and progressing beyond the event may be critically impaired.

As time passed in the hospital, I realized that once I understood some fundamental words used in the cardiac community, I could have decent conversations with another heart attack victims and medical staff. Why wasn't I just handed an FAQ pamphlet with common words and definitions upon my arrival into the cardiac wing? If that had been the case, I would have been able to absorb what the medical staff was saying from the very beginning hours, converse more easily with my cardiologist, and begin to comprehend what happened to me. Instead, victims are left on their own to put the pieces of their puzzle together, in another language.

The hallway conversations with other cardiac patients continued with frequency and their unique stories unfolded. Another new friend told me he had been suffering with what he thought was indigestion one evening and all through the night. Nothing he did seemed to relieve his symptoms. He still felt this "indigestion" the morning after a fitful rest. He got up and was getting ready for work when debilitating pains shot up his neck, across his chest, and down his left arm. He couldn't breathe, lost his balance, and then fell to the floor. His wife called 911 and the next thing you know, he was on the operating table.

This was such heavy and sad news for me to hear, yet at the same time, I knew this story was very common. The more patients I talked to, the more it seemed that many of their stories started with indigestion-type symptoms, which is really pain caused from a blockage in an artery. Why don't we all know this? If a person has unresolved indigestion, it could actually be pain from a blocked artery. I will also ask again: What kind of heart attack did you suffer from? Knowing specifics is vital to your recovery plan and healing trajectory. Unfortunately, most times it is only when we ask very specific questions to medical staff that they share detailed information. If we don't ask, much is not explained. Here are the three types of heart attacks. What are the specifics to your unique event? Is it even listed here?

1. ST-segment elevation myocardial infarction (STEMI, known as the classic heart attack)

2. Non-ST-segment elevation myocardial infarction (NSTEMI)
3. Coronary spasm or unstable angina

HEART ATTACK SYMPTOMS

Heart attacks are not always like what's on TV, where a guy grabs his left arm in pain and falls to the ground. There are many signs and symptoms of a heart issue or heart attack that everyone needs to be educated on for ourselves, our families, and friends as well. If you or a loved one has had a heart attack, you have been forced to become intimately familiar with symptoms. If you are lucky enough not to have anyone in your circle without a heart condition, it still remains critical to educate yourself and those you love on heart attack symptoms. Here they are as a common list from the American Heart Association (AHA), Center for Disease Control and Prevention (CDC), and other well-respected institutions:

1. *Chest pain, pressure, and discomfort.* Excruciating painful pressure, severe tightness, clenching feeling across the chest, extreme heaviness on the chest, and/ or crushing pain. Many victims mistake these symptoms for a form of indigestion, but the crushing heaviness is undisputable, hence the phrase "elephant on one's chest."
2. *Sweating.* Intense, uncontrollable, profuse sweating sometimes coupled with pallid face color. This can be difficult to surmise for a woman who is going through menopause and has hot flashes.
3. *Shortness of breath.* Could be mistaken for

oncoming allergies, or a head or chest cold, but most people experience having an undeniably difficult time breathing, especially when exerting oneself, for example, when taking the stairs.
4. *Indigestion and/or stomachache.* This is misidentified chest pain which may be angina pain caused by blockages, with an oncoming heart attack.
5. *Abnormal or irregular heartbeat.* Especially when accompanied by dizziness and/or fatigue. Often confused with panic attacks.
6. *Pain in throat or jaw.* This can be a constant pain or a sharp, sudden pain before or during the heart attack. It is a very unusual sensation, one that you have never had before.
7. *Exhaustion.* This is not your normal tiredness. This is above and beyond. You can't do the same things you used to do, like walk or hike, or simple chores without feeling exhausted. Even vacuuming or other normal household duties can be difficult to manage. You want to nap a lot.
8. *Dizziness and nausea.* Feeling off-balance, or like you are going to fall suddenly for no reason, with lightheadedness for no reason.
9. *Anxiety along with insomnia.* When we have decreased oxygen in our systems due to decreased blood flow from blockages, we have difficulty resting and falling asleep. This naturally feeds into our anxiety. (These alone are not indicative of an oncoming heart attack.)
10. *Radiating pain.* This is pain that has not been experienced before but instead what is called "new pain," unfamiliar sensations or tingling in

our arms, across our chests, up our necks, or around your shoulders.

Heart attack symptoms can be intermittent or constant. They can last for days, weeks, or months, and that is definitely what happened to me. Heart disease is commonly and medically referred to as cardiovascular disease. I use these terms interchangeably in this book. According to the CDC, only 27 percent of Americans know what the symptoms of a heart attack are, so when they are happening, they either deny it or don't have the knowledge to know what is happening in order to take the proper call to action.

The women I talk to who have had heart attacks describe their experience a little differently than men do. First of all, it's important for me to point out that most women are used to recurring pain. We have it monthly for much of our lives. We give birth to children and we tend to deal with headaches and other uncomfortable sufferings on a regular basis. I am suggesting that our tolerance for pain is different than men's – not necessarily higher, but definitely different. I want to offer up that we women tend to be mindful of our pains and then *push through* them. We do this because we are accustomed to doing this monthly. We do this because we have families to take care of, jobs to go to, houses to keep clean, and meals to put on the table. We do this because that is the behavior that we witnessed from our grandmothers, aunties, mothers, and sisters. I am sure there is research out there on the subject of women pushing through life when feeling like shit, but I am not here to debate that specific point. Instead, I am suggesting that many women experience heart attack symptoms long before the heart attack event but ignore them, work through them, push them away, or mislabel them. Also, many women are repeatedly told by their doctors that when they are feeling symptoms, it is due to stress, our hormones, or our cycle, and that we need to relax more (a subject not to be tackled here). As a result, we don't go to the doctor when we need to because we feel that we can figure it out or push through it until we are on the other side. The unfortunate part of this ingrained behavior is that some symptoms are really indicators leading to a point of no return.

HEART ATTACK SMACK

A heart attack strikes a person in our country every forty-three seconds, according to the AHA. Heart disease is the number one killer of women in the U.S. and globally. *The number one killer of women.* Not cancer. Not anything else.

I will emphasize that if you or a loved one write off your symptoms as being something else or less than life-threatening, it could be a very dangerous decision. Here is a list of what some of my clients have shared as excuses that they told themselves prior to having their heart event: "I had a cold, that's why I was tired beyond belief;" "I was working too many hours, that's why I was exhausted and felt like crap;" " I kept sleeping wrong on my pillow, that's why my neck hurt;" "My period was coming on, that's why I felt like crap despite the sharp pain in the middle of my chest and what a weird place to have pain during my period;" or, "My symptoms were flu-like, but no need to see the doctor," *even though they have lasted for a month*. And then, to add to very unfortunate compilations, our reasoning becomes convoluted. We are short of breath, so we feel our allergies are coming on, or we are dizzy, so we must be dehydrated. To top it off, we tell ourselves, "I know my body best and whatever this is will go away. I just need to rest, turn down the stress, and keep busy." Keep this list handy and add to it based on your event experience.

My new hallway walking buddy was still exhausted and sore beyond belief in his chest, shoulders, and upper back, and the area where his healthy vein was taken for the bypass was tender and painful.

"They say I have 'Pumphead,'" he shared with me, late on day two of my stay. I looked at him in dismay. *He must be on some new drugs,* I thought. I had no idea what this meant and had never heard of this word before. It sounded like something from the World Wrestling Federation, like a Hulk Hogan slogan, but I was still in Cardiac-ville, with no idea what many words meant. Every day I was still being bombarded with long, scientific words or foreign acronyms by the medical staff. Now my hallway buddy was doing it too. I wished my kids would hurry up and get there. They would be my interpreters for this new, scientific language being tossed around in this unknown culture I'd landed in. I shook my head at my hall-mate, showing sympathy, and kept walking around the nurse's station in a circle. It was best to drag the IVs with purpose, ensure your butt isn't hanging out, and listen for the lullaby to play on the hospital speaker system, announcing another baby was born.

Pumphead. Pumphead. According to Google, Pumphead is a name given for a condition a patient can experience after open-heart surgery. Described in more detail, during post-surgery, the patient has trouble remembering, slower mental processing, moodiness, depression, and difficulty focusing. Pumphead is common for those who have had coronary artery bypass surgery, a specific kind of surgery for people whose arteries are too narrow. As a result, the blood flow to the heart is impacted. You would not think that heart surgery affects the brain, but it does. In chapter

5, Light Science, you will learn much more about the brain-heart connection.

Stressors are put on the brain during and after heart attacks or surgeries. This stress is derived from many sources. Here are some: medications, sleep deprivation, inflammation, blood clots that develop, lack of oxygen, or dehydration. Over time, a person's blood-brain barrier can be impacted if their heart arteries are too narrow. The blood-brain barrier is normally a healthy function that protects our brains from foreign substances. When arteries are uncommonly narrow, foreign substances that would *not* normally pass through the blood-brain membrane are given a free pass. As a result, a person suffers from chemical changes and cognitive impairments. Now I started to understand Pumphead a little bit more, and my mind was literally blown from learning about this brain phenomenon.

This became my first exposure to and realization of the mind-brain-heart connection and in looking back, I truly believe it was a major catalyst for me to write this book. I was starting to realize just how much I did not know about my heart, my event, and my body's influence on it all. I felt helpless and was left in a state of despair, which was not a common feeling for me to have. I prided myself on learning, growing, and being in the know, then here came this Pumphead word, one of many that came rushing at me. Fascinating stuff indeed, but God, I hoped my brain was OK. Shit, was it? I needed to take some serious action in the direction of fully educating myself about my heart and brain, and I hoped it wasn't too late.

I continued lying in bed trying to reconstruct: *How exactly did I get here again?* I began retracing the events in my life just a couple of days before my heart attack, looking for clues that I should have been mindful of. This is what you need to do as well, when ready, by yourself or with someone. Review what happened the week or so prior to your heart event for a complete understanding. You may even realize that you need to go back even further than one week. You will learn from this. It will help you identify what you missed, or possibly what other people are missing, that were your unique pre-heart attack signs and symptoms. Below is an example of the events and symptoms I experienced in the days leading up to my heart attack, and most importantly, how I kept making excuses for them and pushing them away. See how many symptoms with excuses I had that you can pick out, and witness how they kept stacking up.

SPARTAN FOOTBALL

Just a couple of days prior, I was attending a Michigan State football game in East Lansing. It started off as a beautiful October Saturday. The colors of the leaves on the trees looked amazing, just as you would expect from a fall Michigan day. I had been under so much stress at work; this would be an awesome escape. I brought my childhood friend Robby with me, another MSU grad who I grew up within my Clarkston, Michigan neighborhood called Birdland. It poured rain throughout the entire game. I ended up getting chilled and feeling miserable. We parked across from campus, which normally would be an easy walk for me, but that day, it wasn't. It was difficult for me from an energy and breathing perspective, but I attributed it to the rain and chilled temperatures.

I was so tired too. I remember feeling like I hadn't slept in week. But what did I do? I shrugged it all off, convincing myself that everything I was feeling was from the stress of my job and the weather. More importantly, I didn't want to ruin my time with Robby because having a fun activity together, alone and separate from his family, was a rarity for us to enjoy.

On the drive back, we stopped to visit Robby's sick dad. At this point, my tiredness seeped into every bone of my body, beyond anything I had ever felt before. Playing Monday morning quarterback, this should have been a sign and clue for me to take some kind of action, like going to a Minute Clinic or maybe urgent care. But, with aches and pains starting along my back and neck, I blamed it on those darn football bleachers and the damp cold. This is what I kept telling myself. Once we were at the dad's house for the visit, I had to excuse myself and go into the adjacent room to do some deep breathing and yoga poses. I was bound and determined to work those aches and pains right out of my body. But this time, it didn't work. The aches and pains stayed with me through the night.

PAINT CREEK TRAIL

The next day, Sunday, I was committed to attending my brother's mother-in-law's funeral. It was a stressful and sad day, as expected from a funeral. I felt especially out of sorts because my body still felt exhausted (not tired, but exhausted), and now I heard myself telling people I felt "out of whack." But hey, I was at a funeral. *Maybe I'm getting sick?* I told myself to take more vitamins and get lots of rest when I got home. *That should definitely make me feel better.* I pushed through the full funeral day like the warrior I was accustomed to being.

When I returned home from the funeral, I went to the Paint Creek Trail to take my evening walk. *This will de-stress me* – again, a hopeful sentiment on my part. I started walking, but every time I took a few steps, I couldn't breathe very well, and do you know what I told myself this time? I told myself that my allergies must be coming on and I brushed it off. I started my walk and stopped, started and stopped over and over again, hitting up just a short bit of the trail. I noticed a woman watching me as she approached from the opposite direction. Unbeknownst to me, a divine intervention was upon me.

This angelic woman was my physician's assistant (PA) from my doctor's office. There she was, jogging toward me from the opposite side of the trail. I couldn't believe my eyes and started to tear up. Why? Because I felt like total shit and seeing her brought me relief. I had walked this trail daily for years and never had I randomly bumped into my PA. It was overwhelming in my present state. She stopped with a concerned look, asking me how I was doing. I told her. I let it all out. Ran down the list of symptoms that I'd been having over the last three days and didn't hold back. She listened attentively and then in her calm, reassuring voice, told me to go to my primary doctor first thing in the morning and get a stress test. She said not to be worried, but that we needed to rule out the possibility that something was wrong with my heart. *My heart? Did she say my heart?* I had no history of or any indications for such a problem. My numbers were all good for years, better than the normal ranges. I thanked her, gave her a hug, and went straight home.

For the rest of the evening, I kept repeating in my head what she said. No way was it my heart. I was in good shape, with consistent activity, and had had blood work and check-ups with my doctor not yearly, but every six months for the last five years. I was committed to my health and swore to myself that I would never allow myself to have issues like my parents did. No way. My actions and behaviors had been cemented in the promise that I would always take care of myself. It's not my heart. It's a sinus infection, yeah, a sinus infection. I lay in bed at home trying to relax, with my monkey-mind wrapped around my sinuses.

You can clearly see that there were so many symptoms, signs, and feelings that kept stacking up against me. You may realize this as well about yourself and your pre-heart attack days. Are we too stubborn? Is there a lack of knowledge? Do we just push through because that is how we have always dealt with things?

MESS INTO A MESSAGE

But back to my hospital bed. I began to realize that throughout my entire life, I had been connecting the dots related to my genetics and heart incidences in my life. Why? Because when I was growing up, my father suffered from heart problems, along with many other chronic illnesses. He took meds for his blood pressure in addition to his heart condition. He saw his cardiologist regularly and after one appointment, when I was about twelve years old, I remember Dad being so elated because he was able to come off of some meds – the artery that was blocked had grown new blood vessels, which bypassed the blockage! "A miracle!" He said. Much-needed oxygen-rich blood was now flowing through these teeny tiny new capillaries, bringing much-needed nutrients to his heart, to then course through his body. He was a new man with a renewed sense of life passion and a little flush to his cheeks. He began to mow the lawn again, took my brother fishing, and seemed to smile more, with that special twinkle in his beautiful blue eyes.

Growing up, I would talk to people I knew who had had heart attacks, parents of friends who survived, about what they did to recover. I devoured a lot of books about heart attacks, all written by doctors. Finding a book written by a cardiologist who had actually had a heart attack was impossible, but there were books written by neurologists who actually suffered from brain injuries. Those were fascinating stories with power behind their words for me, because the authors had the credibility of the actual medical experience. Books available on the heart focused on the medical aspects of cardiology – how to improve the function of your heart, strategies to prevent heart disease, and how to maximize required lifestyle changes. What about a book for the tsunami of emotions and feelings victims drowns in after their heart attack? What about how lives are turned upside down with the struggle to get things back in order? How can survivors learn to trust their bodies when dealing with the feelings of overwhelming fear, numbness, and anger associated with this new lack of confidence?

I lay in the hospital bed, finally hearing the merciful voices of my kids coming down the hall toward my room. A huge smile came across my face. I will write that book, that book about heart attack recovery, with all its emotional twists and turns, written by a normal, everyday person who had a heart attack and now struggles with how to live life. I started journaling right then and there about all that I was going through. In those moments, I felt massive amounts of relief because I had a new, higher purpose. Maybe I did have a heart of gold, as my childhood friend used to tell me.

Two days after my heart attack, I focused on this new purpose of turning my mess into a message. I realized that my heart attack needed to help a lot of people. I survived for a reason, just as you have, and my event would serve others. I would share my experiences, struggles, and the importance of genetic predispositions, create a faithful healing process and communicate how to make healthy lifestyle changes. This book will help propel victims into making their way to an abundant future. My new life passion became heart attack survivorship.

The next day, I contacted my boss and resigned from corporate America after giving it much of my last thirty years of life.

3

HOW TO READ THIS BOOK

"The more that you read, the more that you'll know. The more that you learn, the more places you'll go."

— DR. SEUSS, *I CAN READ WITH MY EYES SHUT*

First of all, I want to thank you for choosing this book. It takes a lot of courage to take action to help yourself when feeling sad, lost, or out of control. If you or someone near you is recovering from a heart attack, you might be feeling these very same things, and don't know where to turn. With this book, you have taken a step to recognize and acknowledge your literal heartbreak, and the critical need to reach out for support. You and your loved ones only have one life to live, so learning how to best get on with it in positive and curious ways is very healthy. Time is going to pass you by, no matter what. The first question to ask yourself is, where do you want to be in three, six, or twelve months? You will arrive somewhere, but where? This book will help you get to the future you desire. I recommend having a journal by your side as you take this heart-healing ride.

At first, after surviving a cardiac situation, you muster through all the emergency medical attention that is required. If you're like me and most other survivors, immediate medical care was accomplished, but you don't really remember the details because you were in a lot of pain and a mental fog. For the next few days and weeks, you are in and out of the hospital, doctor appointments, and procedures. It is normal not to remember everything that happened and when it happened, let alone what is expected to happen next. Your doctors told you many things, most likely have given you a lot of meds, took you to the cath lab, did tests and possibly surgeries, and then released you again from the hospital with a stapled pack of instructions on what to do. This is completely overwhelming. In the paper pamphlet they gave you, you learn about any restrictions you need to respect, like a requirement to stay home and rest, to not return to work yet, or lifting no more than a gallon of milk. Cardiac rehabilitation may be discussed as an option. There may also be limitations on what kind of activities you can or cannot do. For me, I was banned from doing any yoga inversion poses for a long time. This sounds like a strange and different sort of restriction, but I could not risk reversing my blood flow away from my heart during crucial recovery.

Much has been left for us to deal with. That's where this book comes in play. It is a step-by-step Heart Healing Process for you and your loved ones to experience, that will get you through the hard stuff in an easy, friendly way. The Heart Healing Process originated from my journal that I have kept every day since my heart attack. It will show you how I successfully navigated my recovery. You're here because the life you had has been lost, and you deserve to live with confidence again. You are starting to realize that you will need to carve out your new, changed life that incorporates ways to accept your body again. You are here, where every other heart attack survivor has been, and feeling lost, depressed, out of control, and stuck is normal, #truth.

Fear no more, because I can tell you that you will get off that couch. You will drive again and leave the house with confidence. Excitement shall flow through your body as you walk the beach, hike a trail, or cuddle with your special person. I've written this book as a gift from my heart to yours, for you to find answers and regain control and order in your life. I will walk alongside you, guiding you through the Heart Healing Process, while sharing my personal experiences. Remember, you are healing your heart both from a physical and emotional perspective.

This book will help you with the suffering you have been experiencing, through specific methods and an order of steps. The order is an organic approach that, from my and others' experiences, follows a common progression toward survivorship. There will be activities and exercises referenced, sometimes to assist you with your healing. Other people's heart attack experiences will be shared, along with what I did after my life collapsed, to successfully move on. The Heart Healing Process will guide you through your recovery, and it can be experienced in four ways.

OPTION 1: READ THE BOOK YOURSELF, FRONT TO BACK, IN CHRONOLOGICAL ORDER.

Choose this option for experiencing this book if you:

- Want to experience this book all by yourself in order to get a grasp on things.
- Enjoy going in the order of a recommended process or method.
- Relish starting from the beginning if there is not a specific chapter you feel the need to turn to right away.
- Are in the hospital for a while and crave moving forward as soon as possible to start feeling some control in your life once again.
- Are at home starting your recovery, and are not happy with what you know or more importantly, what you don't know.
- Need to be motivated and create some momentum to start moving toward your healing phase.
- Know that you need to educate yourself about this heart attack that broke you and your life, but don't know where to start.
- Or, maybe you are a support person or a caregiver for a heart attack victim and want to understand what they are going through, to increase your empathy and compassion skills, which will ultimately help them.

OPTION 2: EXPERIENCE THE BOOK WITH SOMEONE ELSE.

Choose this option for experiencing this book if you:

- This approach can be a wonderful experience! If you have a caregiver or main support person(s), reading this book together can be a joint healing adventure. You can be read to while you rest in

bed, or you can take turns reading to each other. Experiencing this book with someone else brings a whole new dimension. It bonds and connects you. A lot will be learned, shared through conversation, creativity will emerge, and possibilities shall arise.
- Or, maybe you want to experience this book with a new connection, someone who has recently come into your life since your event or because of your event. What a wonderful way to get to know each other, get close quickly, and develop trust.
- If you are in cardiac rehab, maybe you have connected with a specific individual or with the whole group that meets in the waiting room prior to class starting. Pass the book around. Talk about it. Share amongst each other, as you are all experts.
- If you have kids that are reading-age and old enough to share with, have them get involved with this adventure. They will learn a lot alongside you. It will give you common ground for conversation, building trust, and most importantly, having the kids learn about their bodies too. Family time and family growth is crucial at this fragile time. Everyone will benefit.

OPTION 3: CHOOSE YOUR OWN ORDER.

Choose this option for experiencing this book if you:

- Have a special need at this moment in time that requires learning and attention. Skipping to a specific chapter or step in the process right off

the bat is perfectly fine. It means that you are honoring a burning need and want to dig right in.
- Are hesitant about starting a book because you normally may not finish a book. Go in the order that meets your curiosity for that day. With so much that feels out of control, picking what you desire to read at the time and in what order to read it feels really good. It's a baby step, but it is still a step.
- Are a caregiver or a support person and are dealing with a specific situation. Go to that section of the book to help you manage that situation.
- Have an overwhelming need that day and you know there is an activity, step, tool, or exercise that you can do to meet your immediate need. Jump right to that section. (This requires that you familiarize yourself with the book's chapters and steps.)

OPTION 4: CHUNK IT OUT.

Choose this option for experiencing this book if you:

- Have little bits of time, here and there, and can only dedicate a short amount to reading.
- Have a burning desire to read one specific area.
- Are running errands and have time in the car, when sipping coffee, or in between errands to read a chunk.
- If you are a bathroom reader, place the book in your bathroom

I wish I could tell you that the healing and recovery process will be easy, not a lot of work, and will happen overnight. I'd be lying if I did. I wish I could give you some magic fairy dust to wave over yourself and your world to turn back the hands of time, taking you to a place you want to return to, but this also is not possible. Start now in being truly honest with yourself because you know, deep inside, that going back isn't possible. You may not want to face your Truth, but it will be found through this process. Allowing yourself to experience a healing process is giving yourself the gift of conscious, loving and patient attention. It is not a black and white situation, nor will it be a pure linear journey. There will be bumps in the road, painful discoveries, and your Truth with a capital "T" will be uncovered.

The Heart Healing Process in this book safely navigates you from your event, through healing, recovery, and beyond. Your inner critic will want to make judgments about your journey. Push them aside. Focus on being real for yourself, being honest about what you have experienced, and ask yourself, as you go from one step to the next – am I really digging deep? Am I really working through this journey knowing that I can have freedom from constant worry about another heart attack, freedom from the negative picture I have painted of myself, and freedom from the guilt and shame that I am starting to feel and carry?

Here is the ten-step Heart Healing Process that we will journey through together.

STEP 1: UNDERSTANDING HEART DIS-EASE AND THE SHAME GAME

You don't just have a heart attack, come home, and go back to normal. There is a lot you will face that you've never faced before, thought of, or even knew about because the details around having a heart attack or heart event are new to you and not commonly talked about. It is here that you will learn about the negative talk, responses, feedback, and behaviors from yourself, family, friends, and society as a whole in response to your event. I will show you how to notice the obstacles you're facing, acknowledge, and deal with them. This starting approach gives you points of reference, a solid place to begin the steps through recovery and healing.

STEP 2: LIGHT SCIENCE: KNOWLEDGE IS POWER

I'll be the first to say that I am not, in any way, shape, or form, a science person. I am a right-brain creative type. My kids can attest to this without hesitation! Maybe you are as well, or maybe you have a medical background, or love everything science-related. Regardless of your background and understandings, this step in the Heart Healing Process will look at some critical aspects of the science related to blockages and heart attacks. My approach helps to ease a heart attack victim to begin uncovering what may have happened to them. This is a start to helping you put together your specific story as to how it happened and why. Knowledge is power and by doing this, you can embrace what has happened in an accepting way and then pull this knowledge forward to help you even more.

STEP 3: TAKING INVENTORY: YOUR TRUTH

Out of all the chapters, this is where the rubber really meets the road, and you learn of your Truth and how to speak your Truth. Take inventory! This was a difficult process for me but after I completed it, a heavy load was lifted and I was able to move forward in my new life with freeing conviction, aligned to my new values and living my vision. It's a tough and painful chapter, but necessary. Why? For many reasons. You will be facing your real, deepest inner self. You will be digging deep to uncover uncomfortable factors that may have contributed to your heart attack. You will be looking for any people in your life whose negative vibes surrounded you and whose shared experiences were void of joy. Taking inventory looks at the elements of a *pre-heart attack* life, then defines and analyzes them through reflection.

STEP 4: STAGES OF GRIEF

In this chapter, the emotions associated with post-heart attack shock and the associated grieving process will be addressed. The very well-known five stages of grief are shock and denial, anger, bargaining, depression, and acceptance. No, you are not going crazy. No, you have not lost your identity. And no, you won't feel like this forever. The fear, anxieties, depression, and other emotions experienced after a heart attack are normal reactions, even though nothing really feels normal. Most victims truly felt like they were dying when their event occurred. This is extremely terrifying and traumatic. According to Dr. Andrew Steptoe, a well-respected psychologist, epidemiologist, and department head of Behavioral Science and Health at the University College of London, having a heart attack or any cardiac event results in having severe psychological reactions. He writes about how common it is to have depressive symptoms as a victim, and the need to travel through the stages of grief. You will learn how to concentrate on your life and look at the stages of grief differently.

STEP 5: PILLAR PEOPLE, SUPPORT NETWORK & GET ORGANIZED

This step is critical for keeping mentally sane, knowing where to go when stumbling around, and getting help to get through a tough day. You do not have to, nor are you meant to, tackle this alone. Staying isolated is not healthy, especially after what you have already gone through. Please make a conscious choice to rely upon a support network, putting one in place with pillar people to rely upon. This will make your heart healing journey a lot less tenuous.

For a peek ahead, one key word here to describe *all* people in your support corner is "non-judgmental." People who judge make you feel like you are constantly walking on eggshells, never knowing when a dagger of a remark will be thrown at you. People that give you judging looks or stare-downs are going to drag you down into their pit of despair. In this chapter, you will learn how to mindfully pick and surround yourself with the right people while walking through the key, instrumental steps to getting organized. I refer to this as "getting your ducks in a row." This is required at many levels: daily routines, post-heart attack habits, protecting critical energy reserves, and reducing stress levels to name a few.

STEP 6: UNPACK YOUR CRAP

This is one of my favorite chapters and steps in the Heart Healing Process because it is about freedom. The results of your inventory process position you to let go of that which does not serve you, with a dose of radical acceptance, thus opening the gate to your awakening stage. You didn't ask for a heart attack, and certainly, under no circumstances, did you deserve one. You have to trust this and know in your heart that when you unpack your crap, you are choosing where to spend your very precious energy going forward, who to share your love with, and to let go of those who hurt or tormented you. I call it "crap" because at the end of the day, that is how I feel about it. I had all this "crap" I had to deal with that wasn't helping me live a fully healthy life. In order to let go, we have to unpack and understand those experiences, circumstances, and people that are not in our best interest. All you have room for in our life now is that which fills your cup to capacity with healing vibes that help you move on. In "Unpack Your Crap," that is exactly what you'll do: Unpack the crap in your life from the inside-out and the outside-in.

STEP 7: RECALIBRATE

By this chapter, you are ready to take the steps of looking at your life through a different lens, gain new perspectives and take action. At first, not huge actions, but baby steps to start with. Creating new perspectives and working with them brings your power back and ultimately gets you unstuck. You will also learn about the Ten Laws of Heart Healing that provide motivation, support and guidance.

STEP 8: HEART CONNECTIONS AND HEALING

In this chapter, you will learn about the brain-heart connection, how it critically impacts the whole of you, and what can be done to keep it healthy. I studied this connection in the neuroscience phase of my coaching wellness certification program at Whole Life Healing. Learning about the brain-heart connection prepares you for recovery and continued healing. From there, we will talk about a more practical aspect of life: your return to work. Then we will dive into fixed versus growth mindset and the importance of seeking out your inner warrior.

STEP 9: PTG: POST-TRAUMATIC GROWTH

What a great place to be in! We are growing now in this chapter, moving forward and on to live an abundant life again. You now know where you will arrive: in a healthy, growth-oriented, worry-free space and time in your life. Your heart will be awakened in so many ways, permeating through deep layers. In Step 9 of the Heart Healing Process, you will regain strong belief in yourself and in your body. The sky is the limit and so is your imagination. We will discuss ongoing motivation and willpower, and how they help you live an intentional, authentic life. Most importantly, you will notice a shift in yourself, life, and your energies.

STEP 10: ON THE OTHER SIDE

Soon it will be time to move through the first full year post-heart attack, to the date when you celebrate your one-year "Heartiversary." What can you do to maintain your new routines, and sustain the processes and lifestyle changes through this first year? I wrote this book to speak my Truth about my heart attack, from the inner lens of someone that has experienced this phenomenon. My passion is for you to do the same, to be able to speak your Truth about your heart attack survivorship, ensuring that you have your healing process intact and then to celebrate with a hearty party. Your heart attack only has the power and the meaning that you assign it. You can change its devastating meaning and instead create a new world with a different perspective, feeling empowered, in control, happy, and in charge.

After completing these steps with yourself or through a shared experience with a close friend or family member, you will be able to move forward in your life with faith, confidence, and hope. I know that you are scared right now and skeptical about the whole world. You have every right to be. Your heart has failed you. You are questioning everything about your body, your life, and the things around you. You stare out into nothing for long periods of time with a wandering mind and a sense of numbness. I know. I've been there. You may be putting your valuable energy into blaming other people or pointing the finger at God. These chapters and steps will help you to take the bull by the horns and march to a different beat.

Has the couch or La-Z-Boy chair become your primary comfort zone? Are you watching hours and hours of mindless TV while wondering, "How did I get here?" I did for a while. Maybe you have already jumped right back into your work-life, right where you left off, ignoring the doctor's advice or not taking the time to heal, filled with fear about doing cardiac rehab. If so, you may be telling yourself that this is the best way, that this is what needs to be done so that you are not a burden to other people, and that what will be will be. I've seen this a lot too. Although this full distraction may feel right at the time and helps us to escape our pains, it is a short-lived strategy and can boomerang, coming back to bite you even worse. There is no getting back to normal. You have to create your new normal, a bigger, better, and brighter normal!

I ask that you give yourself the gift of not only reading this book, but the space and time in which to experience it. It can be frightening because you will be facing what happened, and not tucking it away, stuffing it down, or putting it on a shelf in the back closet. If you choose not to take the time to heal emotionally and physically, you may be having to deal with Post-Traumatic Stress Disorder (PTSD) and depression down the road. A friend of mine had her heart attack at night, while she was sleeping. She woke up in a full shock mode, not knowing where she was or what was happening. Her husband called 911 and she got to the hospital in time. After the hospital visit, she returned to her life as it was and didn't talk about what happened to anyone. But soon, she started having recurring nightmares. Her doctor told her she was experiencing PTSD. By leaving her pain behind, covering it up, and not facing it head on, it demanded to be heard and dealt with through her subconscious. I don't want something like this to happen to you or your loved one.

You can get to the other side of this painful time. You can make your way through and into a new life, prioritizing your health and looking at your heart through a new lens of love, light, awe, and gratitude. Trust yourself, and that is with a capital T.

STEP 1 – UNDERSTANDING HEART DIS-EASE AND THE SHAME GAME

"If you want to know who your tribe is, speak your truth. Then see who sticks around. Those are the people who get a spot in your blanket fort."

— NANEA HOFFMAN

When you come back home after your event, you will start to experience a mixture of positive support and negative talk and behaviors from family, friends, and society. There will be obstacles to face and you may be feeling some guilt or shame. On top of that, there may be a feeling of loss if those you expected to be there for you don't show up at all. In this chapter, we will dismantle those feelings of heart dis-ease and the society-imposed guilt and shame, and explore ways of overcoming them.

EMBARRASSMENT

For several months after my heart attack, I couldn't tell anyone outside of a few close family members and my BFF girlfriend Geri about what happened. I felt helpless and the words "I had a heart attack," still would not roll off my tongue. Maybe you feel this way too. Why is it like this? Because we suffer from shock, shame, and guilt, and our whole life has changed. Where are the tribes you used to belong to? Where are the people that you saw every day, the places you used to frequent, and the things you used to do? Your tribes changed right before your eyes after a heart event, and the norms and expectations of your own behaviors do too.

From a social perspective, you don't know yet where you belong. It is a time for reflection, to say the least. You feel the changes taking place all around you, the social changes toward you as well as how you now act. I'm here to tell you that it's OK. It is exactly where you need to be because you have been stretched so far beyond your capacities to even be able to participate in mainstream life.

You will struggle and rightly so. You are where you are for as long as it takes you to journey through. There is no stopwatch or timer. The shock and denial of how this happened is painfully real and may result in a feeling of embarrassment when people ask what happened. *How do I answer? Do I open up?* Hesitation is your response and will be your protective friend for a long time. You will hesitate to share until you are sure about it yourself. My favorite go-to response was, "I had a health setback," quickly followed up with a new topic to converse about.

In times when social media has invaded every nook and cranny of our daily lives and society encourages us to completely disconnect from one another, it wouldn't surprise me if you have been curled up on your couch isolating since having your heart attack. You may be lonely, continuing to hide what happened. Or, as I mentioned before, maybe you went right back to work, trying to act like nothing happened. Why is it that you push away this very terrifying event? What just happened to you was epic, life-changing, and major, and yet the irony is that you can't speak of it. Do others have a low tolerance for hearing about this particular health setback? Indeed, it is difficult for others to comprehend, because we look perfectly OK on the outside, but we aren't on the inside. These are all very real questions. Let's try to dismantle these feelings and find some answers in understanding this heart dis-ease.

THE #1 KILLER WITH A STIGMA

Heart disease creeps up on a person, coming out of nowhere scaring the shit out of the victim, just like any other critical condition. Yet, the heart attack survivors I talk with agree that heart attack victims don't receive the same type of compassionate sympathy that victims of other critical illnesses do. People and society often attach a stigma to heart attacks, which adds to making them largely misunderstood. A stigma is a mark of disgrace, and this is a feeling many of us survivors experience, unfortunately. Let me explain.

Most people fighting serious illness receive sympathy and compassion from many avenues. However, most heart attack victims encounter much more blame, judgment, and exclusion than the former. Many heart attack victims feel that they are judged if they were overweight, blamed for not exercising enough, ridiculed for not being on a plant-based diet, and questioned for not going to the doctor often enough. Another reaction often received is, "Weren't you managing your stress?" It is quite obvious from these judgmental common reactions that there is a stigma attached to having a heart attack – a mark of disgrace. Even though the statistics demonstrate that cardiovascular disease deserves just as much, if not more, of our attention as other serious diseases like cancer, heart attack victims don't seem to be getting the message. Why is that?

According to the CDC, in the U.S. alone, 735,000 Americans have heart attacks every year, with 525,000 being first-time heart attack victims. Cardiovascular disease is most likely found to be the culprit. Heart disease, not breast cancer, is the number one killer of women globally, and more women than men die from heart attacks, according to the AHA. When doctors talk to women about breast cancer, women get emotional, interested, and involved. But when doctors talk to women about heart disease, women are not as engaged, says the AHA. The reality is that one out of every eight women will get breast cancer while *one out of every three women will die of a heart attack*. Maybe there is a difference in how doctors approach these two very different, yet similar health concerns with groups of patients.

Is it fair to assume that a heart attack victim should have exercised more, eaten a plant-based or Mediterranean diet, been closer to the optimal BMI, or should have seen their doctor more along with managing their stress? No, no, it is not. A person would not make these assumptions or ask these questions of someone battling cancer or other diseases. You meet them with sympathy, helpfulness, and positivity. Why are heart attack victims so often denied this courtesy then?

We now know that many heart attack victims were the epitome of excellent habits and health when they suffered their event. If a victim is asked any questions about their heart attack, they can simply and safely respond with the lengthy, but real response: "Yeah, maybe my risks would have been significantly reduced if *all* the heart disease risk factors were addressed *consistently* throughout my entire life, but the power of genetics and the impact of chronic stress plays a role too." Who wants to say that?

Let's look at the case of Bob Harper, a famous, globally-known fitness trainer.

FIT AS HELL

Harper is a globally-known health and fitness expert, plus the *New York Times* best-selling author of many books, including *The Skinny Rules, Super Carb Diet*, and *Jumpstart to Skinny*. As a celebrity health nut, Harper was also the host of the successful show, *The Biggest Loser*. If you read any articles about him, you will quickly see that Harper was always known as the workout and good-diet guy, fit as hell and a picture of great health in many people's eyes. But, in February 2017, at age fifty-one, when Harper was at his gym working out, he went into sudden cardiac arrest out of nowhere. He collapsed to the floor, unconscious. He was beyond blessed and lucky that there was an automated external defibrillator (AED defibrillation paddles) nearby, plus a doctor in the house, who shocked him three times to bring him back from death. Gym personnel went immediately into action and called 911.

Harper told Savannah Guthrie in an exclusive interview on *TODAY* on Tuesday, April 3, 2017, "I was in full cardiac arrest. My heart stopped. Not to be dramatic, but I was dead. I was on that ground dead. I had what they call a 'widow-maker.' It was a six-percent survival rate and the fact that there were doctors in the gym when I had the heart attack saved my life." He woke up two days later, very confused in the hospital. "It was super scary for me because I woke up and I was so confused. I was like Dory from *Finding Nemo* because I had this short-term memory, so I was reliving the heart attack over and over again." They went on to talk about how weeks later, when he returned home, he went into a depression and had an identity crisis. Had he been alone at home, like many of us are, he would not have made it. With the incredible advances in cardiology treatment therapies, his life was saved. As I read more about him and his heart event, I learned that Harper believes that genetics played a big part in his cardiac arrest, along with his paleo diet, which is fraught with animal protein.

One of every two men in the U.S. will develop heart disease, according to Martha Gulati, chief of Cardiology at the University of Arizona, due to the standard American diet. From a family history perspective, Harper's mother died prematurely at the age of seventy, from a sudden heart attack that was unaddressed and unexplained. It is quite possible that Harper had a heritable factor of heart disease. That coupled with his very high animal protein diet led to the formation of arterial plaque.

Here is an interesting perspective too, reflecting back on the previous chapters where I talk about being in a fog, not knowing everything for a while, and being confused. Harper goes on to say, "I was told information incrementally. So, I wasn't told that I actually had a cardiac arrest and died until I saw my file. When I found that out, it was a lot of info to take in. I've always been a person that was so driven and type A and I have my routine, which I love, and when all of that was taken away from me and my whole identity of fitness was taken away, I went through an identity crisis. I didn't know who I was and it became a journey for me. I was going through this new life of mine and having to rediscover different sides of me. It was really hard. It was really emotional and I went through a lot of depression because of it."

Harper turned his mess into a message. He continues to inspire audiences nationwide to go get fit, along with having healthy diets. He started his own heart attack survivor organization: Survivors Have Heart. He also remains passionate about the emotional recovery part and how that is what really helps us to evolve and move on in life. You have to put together the pieces of what happened to you, like a jigsaw puzzle for healthy healing. It doesn't happen overnight. It can take weeks, months, and sometimes longer. Be your own full health advocate and detective. Look for clues. Find evidence. Organize data and assemble your own heart attack story. Action brings control, empowerment, and eventually acceptance and solace to your situation.

HEART HEALTH

120 million Americans already have multiple risks that can develop into heart disease. What can a person do to battle this ensuing development? What are the things to stick to that will significantly reduce a person's chance of developing heart disease? They are known as Life's Simple Seven, but I turned them into Heart Health Top Ten by adding three more that I learned about in cardiac rehab:

1. Keep low blood pressure.
2. Control cholesterol. High cholesterol is a risk factor.
3. Maintain a healthy body weight. Abdominal obesity is a risk factor.
4. Keep low blood sugar to avoid diabetes.

5. Be active, with a lot of daily movement versus a sedentary lifestyle, which is a risk factor.
6. Eat a heart-healthy diet. The typical American diet lacks vegetables and fruits.
7. Don't smoke, or quit smoking. Smoking, in any way or kind, is a huge risk factor.
8. Develop an ability to deal effectively with stress, which is a negative and harmful psychological factor.
9. Very low alcohol intake, if not total abstinence.
10. Emotional well-being: positive emotions in your life feeds into positive heart health, including laughter and having love in your life.

Only three percent of the U.S. population does all nine, consistently. For example, Bob followed most of these critical habits consistently, but since his event, he learned that he had a hereditary condition that led to his near-fatal event. His condition causes higher levels of a particle in his blood called lipoprotein to be produced, which forms plaque build-up against artery walls. Science and technology, the field that my sun-son Dalton is in, can be of real help to all of us when trying to uncover the "why." Uncovering the "why" is imperative for you to learn, change, grow, and move on. If you learn that genetics plays a strong role, this will be a relief because you can then point to something beyond your control that was a part of causing your attack, something bigger than yourself was part of triggering your nightmare. Knowledge is power.

BLAME & SHAME

Dr. Wexelman from the AHA says that as jarring of an experience as a heart attack can be for a person, it does not have to be a death sentence, it's actually quite the opposite. "The first misconception is that if you've had a heart attack, it's the end of your life," he says. "It's actually the beginning of a better, healthier life. There is nothing to say that you can't do the same things as before, but you have to do it appropriately."

That begs the question: How the hell did this happen to you and why do you feel blame and shame? The easy and direct answer is: It happened because heart disease is an equal opportunity killer. No one is one hundred percent immune to heart disease. You feel embarrassment and shame because after you got over the shock and admitted to yourself what happened, you blamed yourself for the heart attack. This is a natural response, but you don't really know all the reasons why it happened. Think of this – given that no one person consistently follows all of the heart healthy ways, everyone has some of the risks, so anyone can have a heart attack anytime, anywhere. That's the main, scary point.

Feeling shame is caused by having a negative evaluation of oneself. You are the only one who knows your risk profile, habits, and lifestyle. You are the only one who knows all the things that you were doing "wrong," such as not managing your stress well or continuing to smoke. You are thirty pounds overweight. You eat too much red meat. Maybe you quit taking your statin, haven't been working out, or your family is plagued with heart issues, so it must be genetics. At a minimum, you know there was room for improvements, and hell no you weren't strictly following all heart healthy guidelines. Own up to the fact that in ways, large or small, you could have been taking better care of yourself and now you have a negative evaluation of yourself, which causes shame.

Again, let's go back to cancer victims. I lost my dad to

cancer and I helped my mother through recovery from uterine cancer. As ugly and horrible of a disease as cancer is, is it fair to say that cancer victims do all the things that they were supposed to be doing to prevent getting cancer? Unequivocally not. Most times they don't even know what caused the cancer. Yet, we hope and pray that every single human that has had to deal with this nasty, cruel dis-ease receives the non-judgmental care required for their best recovery, and to not feel shame.

Does this hold true for lung cancer patients, who were smokers? I offer up to you that smokers who succumb to lung cancer land smack in the middle of the judgment-zone, equivalent to what many heart attack victims can feel. Smokers, who get lung cancer like my dad did, many times are made to feel like they deserve it because they should have "known better" and not smoked. They should have made better choices. Where is their cast to show off their injury? Where is their bandana to cover a shaved head? You can't see their disease, just like you can't see heart dis-ease, yet society is ready to judge what their eyes cannot see. It really hurts when friends, family members, other loved ones point the finger blaming a heart attack victim because they didn't eat right, gained weight, et cetera. Do you see what games can be played when people judge without being fully educated? No one ever asks to be sick. No one asks for a heart attack, and definitely no one wants to feel ashamed.

According to Helen Block Lewis, the well-known and respected founder of Psychoanalytic Psychology, "Shame is one's own vicarious experience of other's scorn. The self in the eyes of others is the focus of shame." You may feel shame from your heart event in a variety of ways. It comes from how you perceive others are viewing you: friends, family, doctors, society, or colleagues at work. More importantly, when you carry shame, you feel scorned, and defined as unworthy of respect. This is indeed a heavy burden: feeling disrespected. It doesn't seem fair that you feel disrespected after having a heart attack, but unfortunately it can be a reality. You have been through a traumatic event that is intensely personal, leaving you feeling vulnerable and out of touch with your confidence, self-esteem, and power.

There is a lot of pain that comes from shame, and it is natural for you to want to reduce it and relieve yourself of this emotional pain. Please be very cautious and steer away from reducing pain by negative means, like self-medication or substance abuse, total withdrawal or isolating, aggression, becoming really argumentative, bullying others, or getting into a resentful mode. These approaches only lead to more negative consequences.

Shame can arise from self-criticism. Here are some words to describe the feeling of shame: self-conscious, embarrassed, self-loathing, humiliation, disgraced, or feeling dishonored. After I had my heart attack, I felt all of these emotions at one time or another. The most vital part of my body had struggled, almost giving up on me, and it was difficult to feel secure in the world, which left me with a full bucket of these feelings. I am sure you or your loved one who had a heart event can relate.

Recurring neglect from your loved ones can also bring about feelings of shame. This gets back to the expectation that certain people will be there to help you through your recovery, but then they don't show up for you. When you feel shame, it is important to understand that it is not your fault. I repeat, *it is not your fault*, but it is your responsibility to handle shame.

Having a heart event is considered a traumatic event with a capital "T." Trauma and shame are closely intertwined because a traumatic experience can easily lead to shame. The combination of both of these together can be a predictor of PTSD. Shame attacks the sense of self, and it is in these moments that you can feel shame. When everything falls apart, a common response is to feel shame, and having a heart attack makes everything fall apart.

Here are some thinking patterns that lead to shaming ourselves after having a heart attack:

- I feel so bad and ashamed about what has happened. I am bad.
- Given the fact that I come from a family afflicted with heart disease, how is it that I never considered that I could be at risk? I'm so stupid.
- I am so embarrassed about my heart attack. I feel powerless now.
- I didn't want to trouble myself with doctors. I am such a burden.
- I wanted to focus on life's other priorities and take care of my health later. I got screwed.
- I feel like crap and have no energy. I am a piece of shit.
- I don't feel safe anymore and very vulnerable. I deserve to feel this way.
- I am overweight and this led to my heart attack. I suck.
- I should have taken better care of myself. It's my fault.
- Why didn't I go to the doctor earlier? I am so irresponsible, no wonder I had a heart attack.

Removing heart attack shame from your life is important for healing. Holding onto shame only allows negative emotions to persist, and this is not healthy. How can we get rid of heart attack shame? What is the silver bullet needed to move you past shame? It is self-compassion and self-love. You need to treat yourself with loving kindness and trash being self-critical. Your head space needs to only have real estate for positive self-talk (mind speaking) to build yourself up, which leads to resilience and makes you feel good, worthy, and capable. When you "mind speak" to yourself, work on having it be nothing less than calm tones, kind words, and soothing commentary. This is what you deserve and need to heal, creating the groundwork needed to spring back and cope with what is going on. Admit and even say out loud to yourself that you have suffered enough, which will be a step in the right direction too. Pull yourself up by your bootstraps with loving kindness and give yourself these gifts for recovery.

When you are really feeling out of sorts, refer to this list of my Heart Healing Sentiments. They will help to bring balance back to you in uncomfortable moments. Add your own to your list of declarations:

1. I am overwhelmed with what is going on right now and this is why I am avoiding "normal" activities and people. I am creating the space I need in order to not be overwhelmed.
2. I am processing shock and trauma and I need to be extra gentle with myself.
3. I am naturally putting boundaries in place to further protect myself as I go through acceptance. Maybe boundaries are new for me. It's good to do. It is healthy.
4. I am dealing with a new health condition. It will take time to accept, understand and learn how to manage it going forward.
5. I am prioritizing my time for me and my heart,

only me and my heart, with me and my heart first.
6. I am tired of having to assure others that I am okay and I will be okay. If I seem out of sorts, I will stop and just tell you that I am having a rough day. I can also say what author Lisa use to say on these days: "I can't deal with things today. I just can't deal. Let me go at my own pace or no pace, please."
7. Needing space and quiet time is perfectly natural and good. I will find my place to go to for my alone time away from everything. This will be my safe space, refuge, and sanctuary for peace.

BE IMPECCABLE WITH YOUR WORDS

I'll never forget the cards that I got from the few people I shared my experience with. They were not the wonderful, uplifting, or humorous "Get Well" cards that you would expect when returning from home after a week-long hospital visit. Instead, they were cards with written sentiments that included things like, "Take it easy," "Reduce your stress," "The clouds will clear," and my all-time favorite, "What the hell happened? Are you not taking care of yourself?" These types of words are hurtful to a person who is already damaged. Please be kind and loving. Here is another, common example of something people say a lot.

Soon after I was home recovering from my heart attack, my friend Robby's sister called and was on his speakerphone when Robby told her that I'd had a heart attack. I unintentionally overheard their conversation from another room. His sister's immediate response was very surprising to me. I expected to hear something caring and supportive like: "Oh, my God! How is Lisa? Is she home? What happened?" or "Are you sure? No way, not Lisa!" Instead, her response was, "Well, this is her wake-up call. She got her wake-up call." What did she mean? Why did she say this? Had I been asleep at the wheel of life and didn't know it? Unfortunately, this is a common reaction from people, especially from those who are insensitive. It's a hurtful thing to say. If you are the recipient of this reaction, I am so sorry and you didn't deserve it. You deserve nothing less than loving, supportive and caring responses. Her insensitive reaction was a reflection of her negativity where she was projecting herself on to me with her true colors showing.

You need to remember that when you get home, you are recovering from being sick and are still a patient. Cut yourself some slack, because it is all very overwhelming. Your life changed instantaneously, and you've suddenly found yourself a member of a new club: The Heart Attack Club, and that there is stigma attached to it. Continue working on relinquishing feelings of shame, and dive into the foundational steps of your healing journey. In the next chapter, I will explain why science will be your best ally.

STEP 2 – LIGHT SCIENCE: KNOWLEDGE IS POWER

"Science is a way of life. Science is a perspective. Science is the process that takes us from confusion to understanding in a manner that's precise, predictive, and reliable – a transformation, for those lucky enough to experience it, that is empowering and emotional."

— BRIAN GREENE, PHYSICIST

There is so much to learn about your physiology that it can feel overwhelming. Where do you start and how much research do you embark upon? The answer is: Do as much research as possible, until you know all there is to know about your condition(s). When you can answer the questions, "Why did I have a heart attack?" and "What needs to be done to avoid another one?" in detail, you have done enough research. You owe it to yourself to take a time out from life to figure this out. After all, a repeat performance is what we want to ultimately avoid. When you face resistance, lean into it and push through until all questions are answered and you are 100% confident in understanding what happened to you and why. Educating yourself *on you* is the biggest priority right now and learning all you can will help you with your recovery and healing.

Research will assist you greatly and comes from many different sources. Much of what I learned came from my peers and the medical staff in my cardiac rehab group. Doctors and survivor support groups were also a great help. But that was not enough for me. I needed to dig deep to find out the reasons behind this mysterious ailment of mine that shook me to the depths of hell and back. Long hours were spent at my local Rochester Hills Barnes & Noble, digging up any kind of available resources that spoke to the anatomy and functioning of the heart, data behind heart attacks, and how genetics plays a role. So many new discoveries were made and new pathways of thinking created. With all this knowledge in my brain and in my journal, clarity started to wash over me. I was able to identify the root causes for my heart attack and this was truly freeing.

You have to dig deep, until you feel satisfied about your "how," your "why," and the "what" related to your event. This action fosters acceptance because once those questions are answered, there is something specific to grab onto. You will no longer be puzzling over a mysterious heart attack, but instead, holding onto reasons. This is taking positive action in your life by administering active participation through research behaviors during a time in your life when control is difficult to come by. The control which you achieve and feel during this step will lift you up and give you confidence. Also, the process of breaking down the walls of the heart event mystery creates powerful, positive feelings, which will lead to long-term healing.

There were many *a-ha* moments for me during my research, "grab knowledge" phase, and that is what this chapter will contain. This data will help answer some of your questions and hopefully pique your curiosity, motivating you to do even more research. Make lists of questions for your cardiologist or material for your next rehab group talk. Much of the info that I learned was really helpful to my cardiac rehab buddies. I realized that not many heart attack victims looked seriously into their "why, what, and how." It was a pattern that I noticed with survivors. Many could not even name the meds they were on or the artery that had been blocked. When I asked them why they didn't dig deeper to understand what had happened to them, the repeated answer was it was too difficult to understand, took too much time, and seemed easier to just leave it up to the doctor. Another common response was, "It's out of my control and I am just doing what I'm told to do." Unfortunately, when this is the case and preventative actions are not understood or taken seriously, the chances of having a second heart event increases.

INFLAMMATION

My first *a-ha* moment came from my adult scientist kids, who both work in the life sciences. They would translate the tough medical stuff for me, magically turning it into easily understood metaphors and analogies that helped me internalize all the information being thrown at me. For example, my son described to me my circulatory system as a roadmap. My arteries became highways, my ventricles, parking lots, the red blood cells, cars, and my "obtuse marginal branch" where I had my blockage, a side street. My cells, blood plasma, and cholesterol all had their directions on where to go in order to keep my system functioning correctly. It wasn't until I had a traffic jam on one of my side streets that it all came to a sudden halt.

Metaphors and analogies made me feel so much more

comfortable with my situation, but my kids made sure that their simplified explanations were also accompanied by solid scientific facts. This was especially helpful when my cardiologist kept talking about "inflammation" as a detrimental characteristic of heart attack incidences. Dalton and Courtney explained to me that the inflammation in my blood vessels that the doctor referred to was not the kind of inflammation I get with from a mosquito bite or a swollen eye. Blood vessel inflammation is also different than inflammation of the muscles from exercise or playing sports, like when I was sore after varsity basketball practice in high school, so much so that I took an over-the-counter anti-inflammatory pill like ibuprofen for relief. Dalton also explained that there is also internal inflammation inside our bodies and in particular, inside our blood vessels. We can't feel this. It remains hidden and silent from us. There is no pain, swelling, or redness that we can see to tell us that our blood vessels have inflammation. Scarier yet, many times we don't find out we have inflammation until we have a heart attack. With this new understanding and appreciation of inflammation, I continued researching it to learn more. Below are key takeaways for me. Go slowly and absorb it at your own pace. Take notes, write in the book margins, highlight, or even make a list of what you want to research further.

What causes blood vessel inflammation in some people? Many things can cause it: smoking because smoking constricts vessels and their critical role of bringing oxygen-rich blood to the body; diabetes because high levels of glucose create toxic LDL which triggers inflammation; high blood pressure because it causes blood vessels to stiffen, which causes wear-and-tear to the vessel lining, both of which contribute to inflammation; and stress – yes, stress.

What causes blood vessel lining damage? One common culprit is when humans feel stressed, hearts start to race, blood pressure goes up, and blood vessels constrict. Blood flow is redirected to the brains to help us think to get out of that stressed situation. This is commonly referred to as flight mode. When we are in flight mode, anger, fear, anxiety, and reactive behaviors ensue and cortisol is dumped into our blood vessel system, causing damage to our linings.

As if that is not enough, the inner lining of our blood vessels releases toxic hormones and chemicals like cortisol, which also contributes to inflammation. With chronic stress, versus occasional stress, cortisol is constantly being released, causing significant blood vessel inflammation. Other chemical reactions are also occurring at the same time, like the oxidization of low-density lipoproteins (LDL). LDL and HDL (high-density lipoproteins) are discussed in a physical with results from your blood work. LDL becomes a toxic and harmful entity that contributes to blood vessel inflammation. This deadly combination results in the development of cholesterol, which is created to act as a band-aid to the lining of our blood vessels. It starts to take up space, and eventually gives birth to plaque. When the plaque ruptures, and a blood clot passes by, the artery is blocked, and a heart attack is born.

You will never hear a person say, I had a heart attack due to blood vessel inflammation. Why? Because no one really knows about it and it's much easier to say, "I had a blockage." People kind of understand what blockage means because they've experienced it in other ways; a bowel problem, a sink drain issue, or a plugged toilet. But now you can explain, at least to yourself, where a blockage actually originates from. This is powerful! This gives a deep understanding and an appreciation for our bodies, what they go through, are capable of, and suffer from. It made me want to eat better, to give my body the food-medicine it needs to fight these negative processes off. It made me feel bad for how I had been treating my body. Most importantly, it gave me hope that I could recover and clean out my vessels. Information is power and lets us visualize in our heads what's going on behind the scenes.

There is so much literature to read to understand about the "inflammatory process" in detail, if you want to dig deep. I highly recommend digging deep and immersing yourself. Therein lie hope and a path to your healing. Keep an open mind while reading all that you can, with courage to face your situation head on. Then, your heart can beat more freely. Stay focused and put in some hard work. You are worth it. You are not lost. You are not alone. You are right where you need to be.

VASCULAR & CARDIO

My second major *a-ha* moment came from my science soul-sole daughter, Courtney. She started to suggest that I use the word "vascular" instead of "cardio" or "cardiac" disease when I spoke or wrote. For my condition, I didn't know if it was more spot-on to say vascular instead of cardio disease, as an example. The two words can actually be combined to form "cardiovascular disease," also referred to as CVD. It took me a while before I really understood the differences between the two. Let's hit this up.

Simply put, cardio refers to the heart and vascular refers to conditions affecting the vessels we have, also referred to as arteries, capillaries and veins. CVD is a combination of heart and vessel disease. But then, there are many heart events, conditions, and diseases that a person can experience. Here are some of the common ones: a heart attack, heart failure, coronary artery disease, PAD (peripheral artery disease), cardiac arrest, and arteriosclerosis. You have experienced a heart event, condition, or disease, or someone you care for has. It is imperative that you fully understand from your medical support team(s) what it is that you have, what the doctor diagnosed and what ongoing conditions you need to manage. If your cardiologist has not specifically said exactly what happened, what you suffered from and how, you need to ask again, or possibly find another cardiologist that is much more thorough and has better communication skills. Do not wait.

Learning about your heart as an organ can also be very interesting. Since it is inside of us, we have to make an effort to see what it looks like. When my first cath lab tests came back, as well as my ultrasounds of my heart, I viewed them with my cardiologist so that he could explain to me what was going on. If you are a visual person like I am, looking at a picture of the heart, or watching videos or documentaries, can bring understanding, which leads to acceptance and pushing away fear. From a simple perspective, these were my takeaways from my research: The heart has valves, muscles, arteries, and a sac around it and these are some of the key elements. Pumping, carrying, and flowing of blood are the critical functions of these parts. When something is blocked or doesn't work right, an event can happen that tells a person that their heart needs attention. Better yet, just like a car engine, cleaner oil may be needed, a hose replaced, or possibly a full tune-up. Regarding your heart and diseases, it's arteries that have blocked blood flow (atherosclerosis), or oxygen that does not flow well (angina), or a heart attack (myocardial infarction).

The list of possible heart diseases and conditions that a person may find out they have *after* experiencing an event is even longer. The list includes diseases that originate from the heart's muscles being weak and/ or enlarged (cardiomyopathy). Valves that are narrow, leaking, or don't close at all (valvular heart disease). Sac conditions from inflammation, too much fluid, or stiffness of the sac (pericardium conditions). Clots deep inside a vein (deep vein thrombosis) and congenital heart defects (CHD), with congenital meaning to exist at birth. Again, it is imperative that you fully understand what kind of event you had, what disease you may be suffering from, as well as what can be done for recovery and prevention. Also, upon hospital discharge, your heart attack severity will have been classified into one of the following categories: low, intermediate, or high-risk group. Make sure you have a complete understanding of what category you are in and why.

BLOCKAGES

Most of us were born healthy. You can say, "I was once healthy. There was a time when you didn't have a care in the world and felt invincible." When was that and when did it change? It is not an exact science, unfortunately, where you can pinpoint an exact time and place, but instead it is a process over time. You can probably pinpoint a few things that changed in your life that caused a decline in your health, but being able to point exactly to the time when you became unhealthy is impossible. It's like living in the Midwest region of America, where there are four seasons. Spring fades into summer without notice and then fall slowly fades into winter. There is no specific day when one season – *poof* – turns into another. In fact, Michigan is known for having all four seasons in a single day at times! It's the same with your health. It is a progressive process where over the years you've had a few bumps and bruises to tend to, along with the occasional upper respiratory infection. Then you start working too many hours, eating habits decline, and you exercise less than you'd like to, and next thing you know, other healthy habits also waver.

Behind the scenes, what really was happening to most of us who have had a heart attack, was that a blockage was forming. As discussed earlier, plaque builds inside artery walls and then bursts off, causing a blood clot to form. This becomes the blockage and blood cannot flow to the heart, causing an attack. The artery has been strangled. Thus, the heart attack appears out of nowhere, but really has been in the making for a while. It can also appear that healthy people suddenly get sick and require life-changing procedures and efforts to pull them through.

Myocardial infarctions (remember, this is another name for heart attack) affect both the young and the old, the seemingly very healthy as well as the overweight and unhealthy. It's a different story and situation for every single person that has a heart event, an experience that needs to be taken very seriously. I had a myocardial infarction of a smaller circumflex artery branch. It could not be stented because this particular artery wraps around the side to the back of the heart and winds around like a small river, turning at blunt angles. A stent could not be surgically implanted to unblock this artery because of the twisting around to the back and its thinness. But I learned that when the catheterization procedure took place, the catheter tip naturally removed some of the plaque that was built up in that blocked artery, which opened up the artery from one hundred percent blockage to about eighty percent. This was a really good byproduct of the cath process. With medical management and implemented lifestyle changes, further blockages can be prevented from developing. I suffered from angina for a few months after my heart attack, but it has fully disappeared. And, over time, my medications dwindled from five to four and eventually to only two, including a baby aspirin. I am very blessed and in a state of good health as a result of my recovery and healing, with no restrictions.

Angina is common in the U.S., with ten million people suffering from it on any given day. It is pain or discomfort in the chest caused by a blocked artery. The necessary oxygen-rich blood is not getting to the heart from that blocked artery, and the pain felt is the heart crying out for more oxygen. For those that have angina attacks, it's best to carry the small, nitroglycerin sublingual pills with you to relieve the pain. Also, stay away from the four triggers: intense exercise (if you are clear to exercise at all), emotional stressors, eating too much, and exposure to extreme cold (under twenty-eight degrees Fahrenheit). If rest along with your nitroglycerin pills do not eliminate your angina within a short period of time, call 911 or get medical attention.

NEW CAPILLARIES

Why did my angina go away? And praise God for this development! It was resolved by my body's miraculous ability to grow ancillary capillaries. These are teeny-tiny little branches that come off of the main trunk of an artery. In my case, it happened off of the blocked circumflex branch artery. They are referred to as collateral vessels, which can grow larger as time goes on. They can also become interconnected, like branches in a tree. The capillaries bring the much-needed, essential oxygen rich blood to my heart, making up for the shortage from the blockage. My body created its own, organic, natural bypass giving me needed blood flow. What a miracle for me. Science is amazing! According to the Texas Heart Institute, collateral or alternative vessels may develop around a blocked artery in an attempt to maintain circulation. For a short while, my heart rate was kept low to not overtax my heart, facilitating energy for the collateral growth to occur. Maybe this miracle is happening inside of you. A chemical stress test can help find these vessels.

The teeny-tiny branch story doesn't end there. Genetics plays a role and further demonstrates how you can piece together your heart problem puzzle. My dad experienced the exact same miracle in his forties. He too had small capillaries grow off of his blocked artery to feed his heart and to make up for the blood supply shortage. This saved his life, because back in the 1950s and '60s, stenting procedure wasn't even on the horizon yet, nor were the medicines that we now have for medical management. These emergency blood vessels do not grow for everyone, unfortunately. They did not grow for my dad's identical twin brother, who died of a sudden heart attack in his mid-fifties. He was under tremendous stress at the time from a recent divorce and his job. His condition was not detected and if he had indicators, they were minimized and not shared with anyone. If he were alive today with these issues, he may have been able to get stents surgically implanted to create the bypass from the blockage(s). From a genetics perspective, my dad, his identical twin brother, and I had similar heart events and experiences. As you will learn further on, there are also other close family members with heart issues as well.

For you scientists out there, there is scientific research that explains what actually happened to my dad and to me in the case of new vessel growth. When a major organ like the heart and/ or accompanying main arteries are damaged because of a lack of blood flow, protein molecules named

VEGFR-1 and VEGFR-2 are released to ignite the repair process. These protein molecules bind to another molecule called NRP1. Together they are transported to the injured location for repair to begin. The healing process is stimulated, and the growth of new capillaries may indeed be the result. What a miracle! My dad's body healed itself and he never suffered from a heart attack! I remember feeling such relief for my father. His organic recovery from his heart injuries let him feel whole again. For more discovery on this, articles by Yale University's Michael Simon and his colleagues on blood vessel formation are published in the journal *Developmental Cell*.

FOOD AS MEDICINE

What else can be done to increase blood flow? Some foods can help to increase blood flow/ vasodilation. Eating as a form of medicine is a wonderful way to mitigate blockages from forming in your arteries, according to Registered Dietitian Courtney Steele George, MPH in Nutrition from UNC Chapel Hill. If we treat our food like it is medicine to our bodies, there are all sorts of amazing things that can happen. Here is a list from the CDC of the top ten foods known to prevent atherosclerosis (hardening of the arteries):

1. *Asparagus* – full of nutrients, fiber, and minerals, and also reduces blood pressure and prevent clots
2. *Avocado* – contains vitamin E, which prevents cholesterol oxidization, which reduces the bad cholesterol (LDL) and increases the good (HDL)
3. *Broccoli* – loaded with vitamin K, which prevents cholesterol oxidization and lowers blood

pressure. Also contains sulforaphane, which helps to prevent plaque build-up
4. *Fatty Fish* – maceral, salmon, sardines, herring, or tuna. Are rich in healthy fats, which clears arteries, plus Omega 3 fatty acids to reduce triglyceride levels
5. *Nuts* – magnesium-rich nuts like almonds prevent plaque formation and lowers blood pressure
6. *Olive Oil* – lowers bad cholesterol
7. *Watermelon* – has amino acid L-citrulline, which boosts nitric oxide production, causing arteries to relax
8. *Turmeric* – main component of this spice is curcumin, which is a powerful anti-inflammatory
9. *Spinach* – filled with potassium, folate, and fiber, which help lower blood pressure and prevent artery blockages
10. *Whole Grains* – contains soluble fiber, which binds to the excess LDL cholesterol and removes it from our bodies

Making these food items a part of your regular diet can improve your well-being along with keeping your arteries squeaky clean. For more detailed information about how food can be your medicine, refer to the appendix added at the back of the book, "Heart Healthy Nutrition."

STATS, STENTS & CATH LAB

Learning the statistics around cardiac arrests can be shocking. They are different than heart attacks. Cardiac arrests don't happen from blockages, they occur from loss of heart function from an electrical disturbance. According to reports from The National Academies of Sciences, Engineering, and Medicine, the U.S. cardiac arrest survival rate is around six percent for those occurring outside of a hospital and only twenty-four percent for those in a hospital. This is shocking. If you happen to fall into one of the statistics that I share in this book, and did not know the statistic prior, it may blow your mind and be intimidating. Many victims of heart events do not survive. But as survivors, please do not cry, for you *have* survived and you will go on to thrive. I know that sounds cheesy, but it's the truth. We are humbled to be in the minority, but we take our second chance at living very seriously and push through to grab life again. Our arms will wrap around it like a tight, warm blanket, filled with gratitude forever. We didn't almost die to live the rest of our lives like we did before.

A woman in my cardiac rehab called herself "Super Woman" and encouraged me to do the same. She shared a lot whenever we were treadmill buddies. When she found out I didn't have stents, like her, she got pretty angry about it and instilled the fear of God in me for not *insisting* upon getting stented. She tried to convince me to get a second or even a third opinion and not stop until I found a cardiologist who would stent me. She said that I was probably barely hanging on, in the grips between life and death, but once I got "stented," I'd be fixed forever. The next time I saw her, she came over to me to ask me if I would go through life with a clogged sink or how long would I deal with a plugged toilet? One thing I was sure of, I wasn't going to deal with her negative vibe anymore. I avoided her. I did not like her energy and I certainly did not need that stress when I was in my cardiac rehab program. Plus, I respected my cardiologist and the decisions we made together. I had confidence in what was done and how I was being treated for my unique set of circumstances. And, if you recall, my body naturally grew capillaries to make up for lost blood flow: my body's own natural stents.

To stent or not to stent is the question. When diagnosed with an obstruction of an artery, there may be the option to be stented, where a teeny-tiny metallic wireframe is inserted through the vessel to open it up and is left there. This is done in the cath lab. The wire is inserted via your groin or your wrist, into the radial artery, snaked up through your arm via the femoral artery and finally to the heart artery. Maybe that's why the definite way to a man's heart is through his groin! (A little humor from the cath lab.)

In my hour of need, my daughter, Courtney, was so excited to hear that I got to go to the cath lab. She had such a positive cath lab experience firsthand while at her hospital internship in Fayetteville, NC the previous summer. What she didn't know is that I was deeply afraid of getting stented. As I laid on my gurney, I repeated little prayers asking God for help through the catheterization process, for the doctor to have steady hands, and to help me face whatever the results would be. A sibling of mine had a widow-maker heart attack the year before mine. Basically, we had our heart events at the same age but one year apart. My sibling had to have multiple stents implanted. As a result, they had to be on major meds to help the body not reject the stents via clotting.

A person can suffer horrible side-effects from these anti-clotting meds and it was these side effects that I was afraid of. Arteries believe they have been damaged from a stent, so blood clots will want to form around the stent and this would lead to blocked blood flow once again to your heart. Medications have to be taken to avoid this clotting, called antiplatelet therapy. I was deathly afraid of having stents implemented and then having to go on meds to avoid forming more blockages. What I finally realized was that these stents helped to save my sibling's life and that they save millions of people's lives annually. Stents allow people to return home, be with family again, return to work, and possibly live to become grandparents. How could I be "deathly afraid" of a medical procedure that saves lives after a person almost loses their life? I was so confused, with a head full of misconceptions mixed with fear. It was less than 24 hours after my heart attack and I can safely say that I was deathly afraid of everything coming at me at that point. All heart attack survivors have to deal with a shit-ton of fear, and where do we feel fear the most? In our guts.

BRAIN-HEART-GUT

Our brain, heart, and gut are intrinsically connected and most people do not realize this. Think about it. How many times in your life have you heard or said, "best to go with your gut," or "I just had a gut feeling?" That is because these feelings are real. We have "gut feelings" about people, things, places, or activities. Remember when you were falling in love and got those "butterflies" in your stomach? They were real, and it can all be explained from a neuroscientific perspective. Our gut holds the key to brain function, which holds the key to our heart. We may even have had a gut feeling about something being really wrong right before our heart attack, but minimized it.

In the neuroscience world, the gut is commonly likened to a mini-brain. Our guts have a network of neurons in our nervous system that connects directly to the brain, and the loop is completed when the brain talks to the heart and vice-versa. The gut itself is the gastrointestinal tract, which consists of many connected anatomical parts: the mouth, esophagus, stomach, pancreas, liver, gallbladder, small intestine, colon, and rectum. There are shared communication lines within the gut-brain-heart triangle. I've often thought about the relationship between my gut, heart, and brain. Upon my first reflection of this relationship, I felt overwhelmed because all of these anatomical parts, or organs, seemed complicated and the ideas around how the three are connected seemed beyond comprehension. But along the way, I've picked up on some interesting analogies and thoughts that make their special connection a bit easier to comprehend.

Within our hearts and guts, we have emotions and feelings that actually start in our brains. Every affection of the mind that is enjoyable, painful, happy, or sad extends to and agitates the heart and the gut, either positively or negatively. I have experienced this firsthand and maybe you have as well. When I was under a very stressful situation or having a powerful emotional experience, I sometimes got angina. At first, I didn't correlate the two, but after my heart attack, I became more mindful of it and discovered that yes, indeed, my brain's thoughts, feelings, and experiences are the superhighway to my heart and gut, because I would get angina in my heart, stomach aches, or tightness in my gut when I was under stress, as my body's reactions to what I was experiencing and thinking.

The other way I look at it is that my heart is to my soul as my brain is to my conscious and subconscious minds. This concept is a perspective with many layers to peel. Think of it this way: all of them together (heart + soul, brain + subconscious and conscious minds) equate to our entire Being. They create our unique experience of being human. It is through their intertwined existence that they chart our paths. Our gut reacts to what is going on, giving the brain marching orders that travel to the heart. But our hearts can override the gut and the brain, commonly touted as "following your heart." Or think of it as the brain being the conductor with our gut being the freight cars and our heart being the locomotive. Modern-day electric locomotives (our heart) can get off their tracks, can accelerate too fast, and can create too much friction, causing accidents, all while the conductor (the brain) tries to stop it. My heart was a locomotive with my gut as the freight car, being bumped along the tracks of life. I followed my heart and loved hard, and I look forward to doing it more.

But how do we even begin to unravel all that is in our brains so that we can have healthier reactions in our hearts and guts? It has to start somewhere, and that is where the 'Taking Inventory' step comes in, as a form of self-analysis that help you discover and embrace Your Truth.

STEP 3 – TAKING INVENTORY: YOUR TRUTH

"You can't go back and change the beginning, but you can start where you are and change the ending."

— C.S. LEWIS

How can a person get to where they want to go on their heart healing journey if they don't understand where they have been? This may sound like an obvious statement, but when it comes to knowing where you are with your heart, it isn't that obvious, because your heart is complicated and so was your event. The most normal place to be after a heart attack can be summed up as "somewhere," and you are somewhere. You know a little bit about *what* happened, slightly more around *how* it happened, and you kind of remember *who* was around to help you. You may even have inner, secret inclinations as to *why* it happened, but haven't dared to share them with anyone. There is a lot to uncover, a lot to put your arms around, and a lot of details to understand. It's critical to point your heart journey in the right direction and this is where going through the Taking Inventory step can greatly help, with no better time to start than during recovery at home. Once the Taking Inventory step is completed, you will move forward with less fear of change and more empowerment, control. and a lot of stress relief.

THE "WHAT"

There is a clip from a show I watched, starring an actor who is recovering from a heart attack. "I'm not in control of anything in my life anymore," he shouted into the phone. "No matter what I try to do, it isn't enough," he shouted again. "Damn, what is wrong with me? I never used to feel like this before. Now, it seems to be a feeling that just looms or bubbles up when I least expect it."

That loss of control is a natural, common, and expected way to feel after a heart attack, because your life will not unfold in the same ways it used to. It is natural – not comfortable – to feel out of control. What happened to you was beyond your control in many ways, especially if it was greatly influenced by genetics. The fact that it happened *inside* of you, to an organ that you cannot touch or see, makes it even more difficult to accept. That loss of control can seep into other aspects of your life and sometimes, when something happens to trigger you, a momentary freak out or meltdown can result. Believe me when I tell you that this happened to me a lot. But there is a lot of hope because over time, there are ways in which you can get control back.

You can always refer back to the Light Science chapter for support when you feel out of control. Remember, the number one way to gain control is by becoming as knowledgeable as possible about what your heart condition(s) are, what happened to you, and taking actions toward healing. You may have successfully survived a lifesaving bypass operation, but that is just the beginning. You need to enter a phase of self-examination in order to understand the factors that precipitated that bypass, which will help you to ultimately avoid returning to another angioplasty, stent, or bypass procedure. This can be accomplished by becoming a critical consumer of information and an expert in the field of your heart health. Become your number one heart healthcare advocate for yourself. Explore the many miraculous life-promoting solutions. Read survivor's stories. Do research. Converse with medical professional about your care and listen to podcasts. Gather all your hospital papers, test results, and procedure write-ups, and check and cross check what you find out from those papers. Focus on continued learning about your condition, keeping it an iterative process, until you reach the point of no more questions. This will take a while, but you are a specialized warrior now, a warrior against heart disease, and the work will be worth it. You will become *the* expert of your body, your heart in particular, and it will feel amazingly powerful. Don't worry if you become a bit obsessive, because it's all good. What you gain in knowledge will lead you in the right direction on your heart journey.

With the digitization of knowledge, coupled with the de-centralization of knowledge, anything you want to know about what happened to you, or are simply curious about, is at your fingertips via the internet. Be a critic when it comes to the articles you are reading and make sure to look at the website sources. Check out YouTube; get hooked on documentaries. Discover what sources are highly recommended for your condition. Bottom line: you don't have to rely solely on what the person in the white coat tells you. Be an A+ student in creating your own health capitol. Fill up an expandable folder with articles, test results, clipped-out correspondences with doctors, letters from friends, motivational journal entries, plus any romantic get-well cards. Make your own library out of medical books written by cardiologists about heart disease. Don't forget your hospitals' online portals to your medical information. There will be a ton of information in there about you that you never knew existed before, so go surfing.

THE "HOW"

According to the CDC, one American dies every thirty-six seconds from cardiovascular disease, and one in every four deaths is from heart disease. Heart disease is the leading cause of death for people across most racial and ethnic groups, men and women alike. More staggering is that forty-eight percent of all adult Americans have some sort of heart disease. I will stress again that coming to a full understanding about how you got to where you are is critical for further prevention, in order to avoid becoming another statistic. There are many tentacles on the "How" beast, and it starts with being one hundred percent honest with yourself. You must be real and true. No sugarcoating data points, nor fibbing or lying to yourself. You have got to speak your Truth, with a capital "T," in addressing issues/ risks you have related to how this could have happened. Respect yourself and keep it real.

Here is the first key question: How have your eating habits been? Have you been eating a healthy diet, or skipping meals and eating junk foods? Was alcohol becoming too much of a standard beverage? Do you even know what it means to eat in a healthy way? Be honest with yourself. It's *critically* important. Wrapping your arms around understanding eating habits allows you to pinpoint negative aspects that contributed to your event. If you were eating a horrible diet, then you know that has got to change, because you understand what happens to your arteries when you feed your body the wrong stuff. If you were dining daily on nothing but junk food along with drinking beers, as an example, that has got to stop. Knowing gives you evidence to support how the blockage happened, where your numbers for key indicators lie, like with cholesterol, and it also supports the needed change. Work with your cardiologist to talk through this in detail, creating a plan of action around heart-healthy diets.

Your Diet & Body Fat

I gained three key takeaways from my cardiac rehab nutrition module: the importance of a heart-healthy diet, the truth about body fat, and the food-brain relationship. First of all, you need to put healthy, wholesome foods into your body to give you the nutrients that it needs to heal. You would never put diesel gas into a vehicle that runs on unleaded petrol. Your body is the same; think of food as your nutritional gas. Nutritious food acts like therapy. It keeps your body healthy, strengthens your immune system, and fuels your body to heal. Therefore, food is a key ingredient and a formidable pillar in your heart health. Refer to the appendix at the end of the book called "Heart Healthy Nutrition" to educate yourself on eating a heart-healthy diet. Even if you believe you had a healthy diet, there is something that everyone can benefit from with further nutrition education from a trusted source.

Remember that eating whole foods is a natural and easy system to follow, a mechanism in which you can help yourself heal holistically. Did you know that many neural chemicals in your brain are formed by the foods you eat? When you digest your food, you are bringing in nutrients that end up becoming the building blocks to having healthy brain function. You need to eat a healthy diet in order to build the chemicals that you need to be healthy. This plays a huge part in creating how you feel, your mood, your attitude, plus your ability to be resilient.

Keep in mind that there is more to body fat than meets the eye. You need to intimately know your unique body, where your fat is primarily being stored, healthy weight, and measurements. Fat is not the enemy. Instead, it's the fat's location and inflammation state which are the risk factors that contribute to heart health. The fat storage in your body is called adipose. There are multiple types of adipose based on location in the body. The fat under your skin that you can pinch is called subcutaneous (meaning below the skin) adipose. Another key fat is called visceral, which is deeply situated near your organs, including your heart. Visceral fat likes to plant itself deep inside of you, like cement poured in between your organs, hiding behind and around your heart, tucked into your liver, and surrounding your kidneys. This kind of fat is necessary for organ energy and keeping your heart protected. However, as I learned from my cardiac rehab nutrition class, fats can be concerning. As an example, my waist was measured every day to monitor my hip to waist ratio, which is a common metric for heart health. If my waistline measurements were not within the healthy guidelines, I received critical guidance and what to do to reduce my fat. Being at your ideal, healthy weight is of utmost importance. Get with a nutritionist or a support person to help you understand all of these influences: your weight, fat storage areas, and eating habits, and make a plan that helps you eliminate any deadly cycles, habits, or behaviors.

Exercise & Movement

In today's modern society, with the use of computers as a main source of interaction, it can be challenging to get exercise in. Because of this, many people have fallen into twelve-hour days of facing the screen. Weeks, months, and even years pass without exercise being regularly built in to your schedule. After your heart attack, it is the perfect time to start anew. Getting into cardiac rehab can be the catalyst to gain back the confidence in your body, or starting to walk can as well. Just like your food, be completely honest about your level of activity. Have you become primarily sedentary, or are you incorporating movement into your daily life? Maybe you've been glued to your desk, your couch, and then your bed.

A regular exercise program is essential to your healthy well-being. You have a clean slate now to create your new beginning. If you are in cardiac rehab, they will give your exercise logs to follow, and will work with you to increase your activity at a slow, gentle pace that is in line with what your cardiologist recommends. They will also create a personal exercise program to follow on days when you are not in rehab. If you are not in a cardiac rehab program, get with your doctor to talk about your plan to get moving. Take baby steps at first, and discuss aerobic activity where you get your heart rate up, as a form of strengthening your cardiovascular system. Your quality of life will improve immensely, and risk factors for having a recurring heart problem will be modified.

With exercise, you will be able to shed weight that has crept up on you. Cholesterol, triglycerides, LDL, and HDL numbers are commonly improved, which helps reduce hyperlipidemia, the condition in which there are high concentrations of fatty particles/ lipids in your blood.

Those nasty particles can be deposited onto your blood vessel walls, creating blockages. You don't want that anymore! However, if you are like me and always have had really good numbers, then this is indicative of there being different reasons why a blockage or a heart attack occurred, and additional detective work is needed.

THE "WHY"

What are risk factors? They are factors that increase the risk of heart diseases like atherosclerosis, coronary heart disease (CHD), and arteriosclerosis. Hopefully, you've been introduced to risk factors by now, from your doctor, other medical staff, or cardiac rehab. If you have not been introduced to them, add this to your ongoing list of questions to review and address with your medical support team. This is vital to healing, well-being, and reducing a second heart event from occurring. Below, I talk about the risk factors introduced to me in cardiac rehab: weight, level of activity, smoking, high blood pressure, hyperlipidemia, diabetes, and family history/ genetics. Stress, depression, and anxiety as risk factors are addressed in the next chapter. The first two, weight and exercise, I have discussed already. The following are the remaining ones, at an introductory level.

Smoking is considered one of the major risk factors, with a person who smokes being three times more likely to develop cardiovascular disease, a major cause of cardiac deaths. Both of my parents were smokers who developed lung issues, among other chronic problems, including stenosis and lung cancer. I educated myself a great deal on the subject. The bottom line is that smoking is horrible to your body and it causes your arteries to constrict and become narrow. Much-needed oxygen is depleted going through your blood and feeding your heart. There is a change in your blood's composition caused from over 1,000 chemicals in cigarettes. The production of plaque is sped up as well, which blocks your arteries. Please work with your cardiologist or cardiac rehab nurse to get into a smoking cessation class to help you through this lifestyle change. Smoking, as a risk, is one hundred percent preventable. Smoking is the number one leading cause of death due to cancer. If you smoke, please get all the help you can to move you through the quitting process: a smoking cessation class, hypnosis, acupuncture, or medications like Chantix and/ or the nicotine patch.

Ensuring that blood pressure (BP) is within the healthy ranges is of utmost importance as a risk factor. Blood pressure is the pressure of blood on blood vessel walls. High pressure damages your walls – this is called hypertension. Your heart has to work harder when your blood pressure is high. There are two numbers to blood pressure: the top number, systolic, which represents the pumping of the heart or the maximum pressure your heart exerts while beating. The bottom number, diastolic, represents the heart at rest, or the amount of pressure in your arteries between beats. The top systolic number can rise with age due to increasing stiffness of the arteries with plaque build-up, which leads to heart disease. Normal range is 120/80, with prehypertension starting around 130/80, or some believe 140/90. High BP can be caused by a lot of factors. Again, gain a full understanding of blood pressure and your specific profile from your cardiologist.

Abnormal cholesterol numbers can lead to many concerning conditions, including hyperlipidemia. It is vital for you to understand the details around your cholesterol profile with your doctor. If you learn that you have too much bad cholesterol, it can build up on the walls of your arteries, causing plaque and then blockages. Work with your doctor to get these numbers to where they need to be. Diabetes can also be a risk factor because it damages the large and small blood vessels, with high glucose levels causing hardening of your arteries. Again, please work with your medical team to completely ensure you are in a good, healthy place with your blood glucose control. If you are not, create a plan and work on it until you reach your well-being goal, and then maintain. Books that I highly recommend reading to help on the subjects of hyperlipidemia and diabetes are *The End of Heart Disease: The Eat to Live Plan to Prevent and Reverse Heart Disease* by Joel Fuhrman, and *Prevent and Reverse Heart Disease: The Revolutionary, Scientifically-Proven, Nutrition-Based Cure* by Caldwell B. Esselstyn, Jr., M.D.

Family history is a complicated risk factor with a lot to be considered. For me, this was tough and emotional to address. I knew all of my life that heart disease was prominent on my dad's side of the family with my dad fighting heart disease all of his life. I did what I thought was right: kept active, checked blood work regularly, ate pretty well, thought I was managing stress, had regular physicals, and never smoked. But this wasn't enough for me. As mentioned earlier in this book, I had lost an uncle, my dad's identical twin brother, to a heart attack in his mid-fifties, his daughter, my first cousin, had a heart attack in her mid-life and one of my older siblings had a heart attack at the same age I did. What's a girl to think? I went to my doctor the month after my sibling's heart attack to have a physical, blood work, and critical tests done, like the CRP (c-reactive protein), which measures inflammation and can be an indicator of heart disease. I was healthy and good to go. Twelve months later, I followed in family tradition by having a myocardial infarction.

GENETIC MUTATION & DNA ANALYSIS

So far, we have taken inventory around "how" it was possible to have had a heart attack, and we've looked at the risk factors associated with increasing the chances of a heart event, including diet, exercise, and family history. Continuing to take inventory at an even deeper level can unveil more crucial information around the how, what, and why factors. After my heart attack, I wasn't able to fully explain the "why" because the risk factors that indicate a person may have a heart attack were in the normal, healthy ranges for me. For example, my cholesterol numbers (a.k.a. my "lipid profile") had always been in the healthy range and stable. My blood pressure was also healthy most of the time, except when I was under chronic stress and it was slightly elevated. So, I had to dig deeper into other, less obvious risk factors, which landed me firmly on family history and a genetic predisposition to something called "hyper homocysteine."

Homocysteine (HCY) is a by-product of protein breakdown. It is an amino acid, a chemical that your body uses to make proteins. Normally, vitamins B12, B6, and folic acid break down the HCY levels you have in your body, but for me, that was not happening. Instead, I had hyper homocysteine, where high levels of the HCY were concentrated in my blood, contributing to arterial damage and increasing my chances of heart disease by twenty percent. HCY is an inflammatory marker, indicative of chronic inflammation. High levels in the blood damage the lining of arteries, allowing blood clots to form more easily, which can result in blood vessel blockages. I learned this through my research, in an older book from the early '90s that I had gotten free from a garage sale, called *The Total Guide to a Healthy Heart* by Seth J. Baum, M.D. In the book, he talks about high homocysteine (HCY) levels as being an additional, accepted risk for coronary artery disease. Behold some truth. I fell into this category and had consistent high levels of homocysteine with my blood work. Now was the time to ask, what did this mean, exactly, and how does this condition happen? So, I went and had a DNA analysis done.

A DNA mutation analysis was completed via a genetic test at my integrative functional medicine office. The results came back: I was homozygous for the c677T mutation in the MTHFR gene (MTHFR = Methylenetetrahydrofolate Reductase). This genotype occurs in about 1.5 percent of the population, and is primarily associated with increased plasma of homocysteine levels, which creates a high risk for arteriosclerotic coronary heart disease because it causes inflammation. Said differently, hyper Homocysteinemia is a risk factor for arterial disease and venous thrombosis. Individuals with the MTHFR gene mutations (aka, me) are at an elevated risk for vascular disease due to chronic vascular inflammation. Admittedly, a lot of this information was a bit over my head, even with the doctor's explanation of my test results. I called the scientists in again: sun-son Dalton and soul-sole Courtney, who explained things to me in a more accessible way.

There it was! Results that gave me the last piece of my heart attack puzzle. I had moved beyond looking at standard risk factors and dovetailed headfirst into a whole other level of exploration, because I was so hungry – no, starving – for new knowledge about my body and heart. It was in the land of genetics, and getting that data helped me to understand the whole picture around *how* I had a heart attack and *why*. I learned how to offset this risk as well: vitamin therapy. By significantly increasing levels of combined folic acid and B6 and B12 vitamins, levels of homocysteine are substantially reduced. For me, this means taking a daily high sublingual B dose and B pill supplements, along with giving myself a B shot every Saturday. Ever since I started this regime, my HCY levels dropped significantly, into the normal levels for the first time, substantially reducing further arterial damage.

Reflecting on this discovery, my gut told me that the chances of my dad, his twin brother, his daughter, and possibly my sibling were born with this same mutation. My DNA test came back suggesting that any children be checked for this mutation so that they can benefit early on in life by taking the measures to reduce this risk. I felt like I finally completed this step of taking inventory. When I look at all the risk factors related, I know what my status is, where I need to improve, how to manage them and the all-around changes to incorporate into my life in order to get the results I deserve. My wish for you is to take your own inventory and answer the how, what, and why behind your heart event by using this step in the Heart Healing Process™. Here is a quick recap before we move to the Stages of Grief:

1. Address + define + be able to articulate the how, what, and why behind your heart event.
2. How does your diet and exercise plan support or not support your well-being and healing?
3. Review the heart health risk factors. Where do you rank with each risk factor? Take the risk factor quiz on my website, Myheartisfree.com, to identify your risk factors, and then work with your medical support team to devise a specific plan of attack to address each of them. Reach out to those whom you care about and have them

complete the risk factor quiz as well. Remember, knowledge is power.

4. Do your research as it relates to family history and genetics. Follow up with additional tests that will help you to uncover answers to your heart situation, like I did – genetics/ DNA testing or other tests.

5. And finally, bring out the inner warrior in you and attack your risk factors with confidence, conviction, and perseverance.

STEP 4 — STAGES OF GRIEF

"Grief can be a garden of compassion. If you keep your heart open through everything, your pain can become your greatest ally in your life's search for love and wisdom."

— RUMI

While I was growing up and well into my adulthood, my mother used to always tell me that I had a special gift of making others bloom. She'd say that when I spent time with a person, if they were struggling, or suffering in some way, my presence and company lifted them up. She saw it when I played on the playgrounds, when I sat at the piano tickling the ivories, or even in a grocery line store doing my random talking, which my kids call "RT-ing." This gift I seem to possess is a little bit magical. I don't know where it comes from, but I am grateful for it. My friend Robby used to tell me the same thing. He would say, "Lisa, you have a special way of making everything be more beautiful, fun and enjoyable. It makes me want to be around you and it really helps my parents when you are around them." I am glad that this has stayed with me through adulthood. It has served me well, especially during times of grieving, or when those I love are grieving.

Since my heart attack, I have thought about this gift a lot but from a different perspective: how to harness this special sauce and use it on myself, to make myself feel special, worthy, and full of joy. I chisel away at it every day, and have since discovered that I didn't need other special people around me to bring it out. All I need is my own self-love. I am asking you to do the same for yourself. Treat yourself with the utmost respect, with self-love, and make your simple tasks and days full of joy *for yourself*. If you have to pretend to be like this with yourself at first, that is OK. As they say, "fake it 'til you make it." But soon, making yourself bloom will become second nature to you.

BLOOMING

When my sun-son Dalton went away to undergraduate college, my mother said to me, "OK, Lisa, now you have even more time to help your daughter bloom beautifully too." I had to stop and think about that, because mom had just had her first stroke and I was mentally gearing up to care for her more. But with four years between my kids, space had opened for a lot of dedicated, loving, and supportive time to be given to my second child. My soul-sole spirit daughter Courtney and I did deeply bond and connect more when Dalton went to college and we helped care for my mother together, all the way through Courtney's senior year of high school.

Mom has been gone for seven years already, but since my heart attack, I reflect on my life through a middle-aged lens and see evidence of what mom used to say about me helping others to bloom. Now, in my time of need, I need to treat myself with tender, self-loving support, to help myself bloom and continue stretching this out to my coaching clients. When you are recovering from life's wounds or a heart attack, your life can feel seemingly in a chaotic mess. The last thing you may want to hear is your mother's voice in your head, but this is what happened to me. I could hear my mom talking about "blooming," while I was experiencing days of feeling trapped in a time warp, one day bleeding into the other as if stuck in the movie *Groundhog Day*. I was immersed in taking meds around the clock, fading in and out of Netflix binging, and being encouraged to eat the right foods. Then, my mother's voice would appear again in my head saying, "Bloom."

A dear friend, who is a nurse, came to take care of me for the first two weeks after my kids left to go back to North Carolina. I was blessed to have this special human being in my life who showered me with care, support, and beautiful get-well cards. To pass the time on the couch, I found myself pulling out other cards I had saved over the years from my kids. Whenever I really needed some motivation, I would take out one treasured card that I received from Courtney. It said, "Mom, you are a budding, beautiful butterfly coming out of its cocoon, ready to burst into the world and show it your amazingness! You have grown so much these past years, no wonder you got exhausted! I am so proud of you and now you must get proud of yourself." Budding, blooming, sprouting, and cocooning – appropriate words describing me as I lay wrapped up in a blanket on the couch, feeling like a crusted old caterpillar stuck in its weave.

Maybe you too are reflecting upon your life, just as I did

during this very fragile time, right after your heart event. Maybe you have some special people who have stepped up to care for you. And, just maybe, you are rediscovering things about yourself that were tucked away in your self-conscious mind from long ago, causing memories to emerge while you start the journey through the stages of grief. Sharing what I went through will help you to know that a lot of the chaotic and confusing experiences you have are not that far off from others who have endured the road to survivorship.

All of what you may be feeling is perfectly normal. Believe me. You have started a very important process that you need to go through in order to recover, heal, and move on to the abundant life that awaits you. This is the grieving process. Don't get me wrong, thank God you did not die, but part of you did: your old life. You will learn to leave it behind, which leaves you space to move on to the new life that you are meant to live now. Allow this time to let go of what was and grab on to the possibilities of tomorrow. Focus one hundred percent on YOU and prioritize YOU. Embarking upon this grieving process with courage, strength and hope will allow you to travel through to the other side. It will feel like a roller coaster sometimes, with some stages easier to manage than others, but getting to the other side is joyous, freeing, and exciting.

COMPLICATED GRIEF

I had never heard of "complicated grief" before my research adventures. Complicated grief, also referred to as unresolved grief, is much more than normal grief. It is when grieving can go on for a very long time, or when more than one major life stressor occurs shortly after another one, and you are led into a stage of complicated grief. An example of this is when a person loses two of their loved ones in a short period of time, like a friend of mine who lost both his brother and his dad in less than two years, and his mother suffered from strokes during that period as well. Symptoms of complicated grief include emotional numbness or not being able to feel or experience love or joy any more. There can be long term depression, a continuous yearning to be back where you were before the losses, and becoming detached from those you really do love. Complicated grief also has intense sorrow that doesn't allow you to return to joyful life experiences or to plan for your future. If you are experiencing any of this, please seek a therapist's help, talk to your cardiologist, and share with your primary doctor so that you can receive the support you deserve. You don't want to be in the stage of complicated grief too long as it will not be good for your recovery and healing, especially because it involves deep matters of the heart.

Aside from complicated grief, what are the well-known stages of a normal grief process? Here they are from the modified Kübler-Ross model:

1. Shock – Initial paralysis from the bad news
2. Denial – Trying to avoid the inevitable
3. Anger with bargaining - Frustrated outpouring of bottled-up-emotions and seeking in vain for ways out
4. Depression and Detachment – Final realization of the inevitable
5. Acceptance – Finally finding your way forward and seeking realistic solutions

SHOCK

The shock stage is horrifying for many reasons. You don't know what's going on when the shock-grip grabs you, and the shock actually started *during* your heart event and then set in. It continues through your hospital stay, feeling like a numbing agent with disbelief sprinkled on top. Yet it is a vital sensation created by your brain chemicals to carry you through pain and suffering. You finally become coherent and fully awake, and the experience of your heart attack is able to start to sink in. You feel numbed again with disbelief, telling yourself that there was no way you had a heart attack. It becomes a vicious cycle of reality mixed with disbelief. It is also blatantly counter-intuitive, because you are lying on an uncomfortable hospital bed, tethered to numerous lines, with a cardiologist talking to you about your heart attack, and maybe you don't believe a word he or she is telling you.

Shock serves a great purpose: it protects you from crushing pains, physically and emotionally. You already endured pain, beyond your wildest nightmares, so how can you possibly be asked to deal with more? Thank you, shock, for being the emotional bodyguard and protector against suffering and pain. Shock is the new superhero that you can trust for getting the job of protection done.

When too many traumatic life stressors happen to a person within a short amount of time, their mind goes into a state of thick fogginess. Thinking straight becomes difficult, memory gets bad, intense positive emotions like love get snuffed out, and detachment from what is going on and from the people you love becomes prominent. For me, I knew I was in shock from my heart attack, and stayed in shock for as long as it took to get through the extreme overwhelming circumstances. It lasted for weeks, but for some it can last for months or longer. Hopefully, you are not jolted back into shock through new life stressors too early after suffering from your heart event.

I truly believe that it is love that allows us to survive our most intense, overwhelming and painful times in our lives. Love from a parent, friends, a romantic partner, a spouse, or children. If you are blessed to have someone who loves you, just one person to help shepherd you through your most vulnerable times, a burden is lifted and your load made lighter. My most wonderful children were exactly that for me: beacons of extreme love during my shock stage and beyond. They possess a deep, trusting, pure love for me that I have only experienced from them. They were God's gifts who mobilized themselves within an hour of receiving my phone call and immediately drove to be at my Michigan bedside. When they found me, I was in a deep state of shock, struggling to make sense of it all.

As you know by now, I am the non-science person of the family. It wasn't until my kids used the words, "your heart has been injured, Mom," that I grasped the totality of the situation. They asked me to think about the approach of a "heart injury" and how healing would be the next critical step. So, I thought about the concept of injury. We pieced together a simple order of events to be able to understand the concept of my myocardial infarction. My sun-son Dalton shared another metaphor: "Your heart, this amazing organ, couldn't breathe for a while. Its critical highways (arteries) were shut down because of a volcanic plaque eruption. During this volcano, your blood oozed around and created a blood clot barricade. As a result, you heart lacked oxygen for a while from this blocked highway and it suffered an injury. Your heart now has a scar from tissue(s) that were damaged from the attack." Isn't that a brilliant analogy to be articulated to a drug-induced patient? In my exhausted, highly medicated state of mind, this was finally a description that made sense to me. Hallelujah! All of those childhood *Magic School Bus* books paid off!

I got to thinking more and came up with other examples. I had gotten a broken finger when I was growing up, while playing football. I also had an infected gallbladder and tonsils that I had to have surgically removed. They were all unhealthy or "broken." My finger healed and the cast came off. My gallbladder was removed, as were my tonsils, and I felt a lot of relief from pain and suffering. However, life did not change a lot for me as a result, nor did I feel like a different person as a result of any of these injuries. With a heart attack, you don't have the luxury of returning to the person or life you had before. You are intrinsically changed, with a new life on the horizon. Shock helps you to absorb this pain, just like the shocks on your car. Shock is your comfort zone from the overwhelming distress from all that is happening to you and around you. Embrace her.

No worries though, as you will not be stuck here. You will eventually move through this shock stage and get to a place where all your efforts will be working toward altering the trajectory of your coronary artery disease, or heart ailments. You will naturally get on board the grief train, which is easier said than done, and ride to the next stage, with this book as a guiding light and dedicated partner. Time to travel to denial.

DENIAL

Your shock will begin to wear off, you just don't know when. Each person is different as they go through the stages. You may notice it starting to wear off when you feel a shift in your feelings that make you want to feel like running away, as I did. Also, hopping on a plane to Florida, or better yet, getting back to my desk at the corporate office ASAP came to my mind. Having an unbearable need to flee means that you have entered the stage of denial, a crucial stage that needs to be fully recognized and experienced. However, running away from the pain, or denying it through distraction by rushing back to work prematurely can be very harmful. You need to take time to reconcile what has happened, as I did. After all, I was still saying I had a "health setback" and still could not say 'I had a heart attack', which are definitely signs of being in denial.

A common mistake made by many people during this stage is numbing themselves through substance abuse. I have witnessed this firsthand with friends and relatives. Alcohol or drugs can feel good for a while, but you are only numbing yourself and stuffing the hard stuff further down. Getting high to get by is not the answer. By doing so, you are physically and emotionally pushing recovery and healing away, which may leave you in one particular stage of grief for a lot longer. It can also be damaging to the healthy relationships you have, and irresponsible because you haven't had enough time to see how your body reacts to your meds. Mixing them with other substances may result in horrible side effects. You may have restrictions to adhere to, or healing to do from a surgery or procedure. Respecting yourself by not running away in any capacity or form is crucial to your recovery. Denying what happened and numbing it with substance abuse makes a person sink deeper into grief and a quagmire of depression.

ANGER

As you travel from shock through denial, a different set of feelings will rush at you: frustration, irritability, bitterness, resentment, sarcasm, and even spitefulness. Notice that they are all on the negative spectrum. A myriad of these feelings bottled up through your hospital stay and return to home, and were stuffed down through shock and denial. When you start to feel them, they are clues that you are in the stage of anger and despair in the grief process.

During this stage of anger and despair, my soul-sole daughter Courtney would say to me, "Mom, you just don't give two f's anymore about anything, do you?" and I would respond with, "You couldn't be more right, sweetheart. I don't give two f's about anything." I also would gladly share my unfiltered opinions on the daily. *Who had time for a filter*, I thought. After all, I could die tomorrow or today, literally. I went through this anger phase where I told everyone exactly how I felt, keeping it real is what I called it. It's unfortunate that this phase coincided with the holidays for me, but damn, that stage felt so liberating!

Sometimes your anger can ooze out of you and hurt the ones you love during this grieving stage, and you might find yourself overreacting to a lot of simple, daily interactions. Maybe you snapped rudely at your girlfriend because she left her personal items on your bathroom floor by the toilet and you just did not like it. Maybe you have an over-the-top angry outburst at her for touching the heat control panel in your car while you are driving. Just like me, you find yourself operating without a filter and not giving a damn, which is demeaning and hurtful to others. Don't worry, you are just passing through this critical step, getting closer to acceptance and healing.

Remember how I told you that we kept it real in cardiac

rehab, because that's the only way that serves you after a heart attack? One of the men I was close to in my cardiac rehab class, fifty-nine years old, shared with me that he was struggling with intimacy with his wife since experiencing his trauma. He used the words "having problems keeping things going down there," and I knew he was referring to erectile dysfunction. He shared with me that he angrily blabbered out to his wife, in the middle of their sensual time, that she had a fat stomach and that's why he "fell short" of the required expectations. You can only imagine how hurt his woman was. I knew, from reading about traumatic life experiences, that this was an example of him projecting his lack of self-esteem and confidence in his body onto her because of his heart attack. He was incapable of having loving, emotional connection because of the trauma, yet he refused to face it head-on. He did not get the help that he needed to work through and to own his shit. I have since learned that they split up, that his wife kept trying to help him, but the further he stuffed his trauma-related issues down and distracted himself from working them out, the bigger the unhealthy wedge grew between them.

Has anger set in for you from the grief associated with losing the life you once had and the body you used to trust? Is anger manifesting itself in ugly ways? If so, own it and get educated about how to handle it so you can keep it in check. Make sure you have enough alone time to process all that is going on, to keep it in check. Remind yourself that anger, resentment, and judging others leaves them hurt, tormented, and lonely. As a result, you will feel shame, guilt, and humiliation toward your own self, everything on the negative spectrum. Reach out to others for help with your anger. Go to a therapist. Talk to your pillar people and lean on your support network to help push you through this stage. The nurses at my cardiac rehab at Ascension Hospital in Rochester Hills, Michigan, fulfilled much of this role for me. They gently talked me through fears, my angry days, and even my weepy times. They were angels. Look for your angels and embrace them.

SITUATIONAL DEPRESSION

Most of us know what situational depression is because we have suffered from it at one time or another during our lives, or we know others who have. It is short term and develops after a person experiences a traumatic experience like a heart attack. Symptoms include sadness, lack of enjoyment, lots of crying, constant worry, sleeping problems, and trouble focusing. I know clearly what it feels like from when I was in a depressive state after my mother passed and sought help to heal me through it.

It is not uncommon to have situational depression after a heart attack, but it's temporary. Seek help at any point if you're feeling depressed, have suicidal thoughts, or if the disruption to your life feels too overwhelming to handle. Seeing a doctor, licensed psychologist, therapist, or counselor is a great help to your recovery and healing. Add them to your support network.

Being sad, apathetic, and feeling "blah" are some of the common feelings of post-heart attack depression. There are many things to do to get you through this stage. I will share the most important with you. First of all, it is very important to rule out that any new medications are the cause of your depression. Discuss this with your doctor. Also, be honest and ask yourself if you are taking your medications on the schedule required. The last thing you want to do is create a vicious cycle of depressive episodes because you are not adhering to your med schedule.

Secondly, refer to the Healthy Heart Nutrition Appendix at the end of the book on swapping out processed foods for plant-based foods. What you put into your body has a significant impact on how you feel and your moods. Try a few experiments with yourself. After you have eaten junk food, see how you feel within the hours following or even the next day. Then, notice how your moods are much more positive when you have been feeding your body nutritional whole foods. For me, when I eat crappy, I always felt like crap the next day. When I eat healthy, I feel strong and healthy. It is pretty simple.

Thirdly, you can ask for a depression assessment that will help determine and diagnose your depression. Work with your doctor on next steps. This may include seeing a therapist, and if that is what it takes to move you forward, put your fear aside and tackle it, because you have a lot more life to live, my friend. Being depressed is more than being in a funk. It is a darkness, and a therapist can help lead you back to light. In therapy, we are face-to-face with our shadows, which are dark. We face them versus running away from them. We deal with them head on, which gives us our power back. We forgive ourselves for what we believe we may have done that contributed to our event.

Lastly, if you haven't enrolled in cardiac rehab yet, do so because this will have a very positive impact on your mood and help your through your path of recovery. Having a lack of any energy is a symptom of depression. Exercises naturally increases our serotonin levels in our brains, which is a chemical associated with feeling relaxed and good. There is a popular movie called *As Good as It Gets*, from 1998, starring Jack Nicholson. When I watched this movie, I remember thinking that yes indeed, we all reach a point in our lives when things feel they are as good as they can get. That's the way it was for my dad when he went through cornea transplants for blindness. It was also like that with my mom, with her series of strokes. I felt that every day I had with them was as good as it was going to get. I learned that people who have had this experience in life fall mainly into one of two categories: (1) those whose days are as good as it gets, and (2) those whose every day is a little bit better than the day before. I fell into the first category for a few months after my heart attack, but after going through cardiac rehab, I quickly and naturally transitioned to the latter group: those whose every day is a little bit better than the day before.

In cardiac rehab class, I would listen to the stories shared in our intimate inner circle before class started. A subgroup of folks were always complaining, making negative statements, and commenting about how life had crapped all over them and that they were making the best of the poop sandwiches they were served. The other group of folks, however, embraced their circumstances, showing up with a warrior-like attitude that was contagious. They *chose* to make as many changes as possible in order to shift their lives in positive, changed directions. It was with these amazing humans that I sought to align myself as I continued to protect and heal my broken heart.

ACCEPTANCE

One day you will wake up forgetting that you had a heart attack. Really you will! Right now, you might think that is impossible, but it's possible and it will happen. When this day finally arrives, you will know that you have truly accepted what happened to you. It has become an innate part of you, of your being, and you are now ready to move on. You will feel more relaxed and motivated to move on with life. For me, following my heart attack, it took me five months to get to full acceptance. I didn't allow time to control my healing, nor did time manage me. There is not a right or wrong amount of time and everyone's progression is different. Unfortunately, I wasn't allowed to stay in this initial acceptance phase for very long. I was thrown back into turmoil from two new traumatic events, one being the 2020 pandemic, and the other was losing one of my pillar people. I was spun back to the beginning of the grieving process, not to return to full acceptance of my newest normal for another four months.

You never know what life is going to throw your way, but regardless, you cannot allow yourself to become stuck in being a victim. Instead, use your power to overcome your circumstance through all the stages of the grieving process. Just knowing the stages of grief and being able to identify where you are in the process is comforting and powerful. I can tell you that I am fully moving forward in an empowered manner, laughing again, noticing things I haven't in a long while, and having special moments in my days. I am much more chill and relaxed, while being excited to be exploring new options for myself, creating new plans, and putting my life back together in a new order.

Here are some questions I asked and attended to soothe myself during the grieving process. They can help divert you from your anger or frustrations:

- What makes me feel good and brings me joy? Let me do this activity.
- Who am I around that eases, comforts, loves, and supports me? Can I be with them now?
- What are some of my favorite hobbies that pass the time quickly for me? Let me start one.
- Who are the people in my life that are positive

influences and lift me right up? I can send cards to them and invite them over for a visit.
- I will rebuild myself by creating healthy boundaries and moving in the right directions with my meds, food, and movement. I'm going to make a list for myself outlining how I will tackle these things.
- I am a strong, powerful person who is in control of my destiny. I will think about my next chapter of life and what I want out of it.
- This is a time of trouble, but I have survived it and I am moving in the right direction.
- As I get my life back on track, I will feel bits of happiness and light peeking through. I will be mindful of this.
- As I get stronger and time passes, I will regain confidence in my body. I will journal as much as possible, so I can read about my journey in years to come.
- This is a delicate process that takes time, understanding, love, and acceptance. I will tell myself to be patient, to love myself, and to be understanding. I will do this consciously every day.
- I will take charge of my future and thrive.
- What kind of self-soothing can I do to help myself? Warm baths, walks, hot tea, listening to music? Let me make a list that I can keep handy.

If you start to think this is as good as it gets, reframe this in your mind. Hone in on your body, your life, and your whole being and consciously decide to not have a doom-and-gloom attitude. You already visited this place right after your heart event. It is not a pleasant place. It was brutal, painful and isolating. Do not repeat being "that person." Instead, actively choose to pursue growth and improvement. This next chapter will help facilitate just that: you will learn how to be your own master builder in creating the support networks you deserve to help you grow and improve.

8

STEP 5 — PILLAR PEOPLE, SUPPORT NETWORK & GET ORGANIZED

"The last time of anything has the poignancy of death itself. This that I see now, she thought, to see no more this way. Oh, the last time how clearly you see everything; as though a magnifying light had been turned on it. And you grieve because you hadn't held it tighter when you had it every day. What had Granma Mary Rommely said? 'To look at everything always as though you were seeing it either for the first or last time: Thus is your time on earth filled with glory.'"

— BETTY SMITH, *A TREE GROWS IN BROOKLYN*

Congratulations on educating yourself on the sea of intense emotions that are washing all over you. Just by knowing about these common feelings after a heart event is comforting. You will move through them in stages in your own time. This unknown territory is hard in many ways, but having a sense of what happens helps you to adapt. You are truly on your heart journey now. Now it's time to take care of your wellness after you were forced to take care of your illness, by getting organized.

There are a number of resources, tools, and things to do to get things organized for when you come home to recover. You may feel scared, alone, or fearful. You did receive a lot of medical information from healthcare workers while in the hospital, but did you get the answer to the question, "How am I going to get through this?" Don't be alarmed, because I know it wasn't answered or addressed in any helpful detail. You will start to take your control back by establishing a primary pillar person for your support, to address things for you. They will become your saving grace. If, by chance, a caregiver or support person is reading this book on your behalf, they have already started taking on the role of a pillar person that they were destined to fulfill for you!

What is a pillar person and what do they do? Can there be more than one? The first time I heard this reference was from my sun-son Dalton, many years ago. He was getting ready to move to Philadelphia by himself to work on his master's degree. He said to me, "I will really miss my pillar peeps" – his very close friends, family members, and those who were a reliable and critical support to him in times of need. He could count on one hand the people that were pillar peeps to him, who lifted him up when he was down, and most importantly, people whom he loved, trusted, and respected.

When you take the time to really think about who your pillar people are, you too probably can count them on one hand. I know that was my case. My five pillar peeps were mostly members from my old, long-time tribe. One of them was on the brink of becoming a new member, if they proved themselves. Over time, that person disrespected me a lot and no longer is a pillar person to me. I don't mean that arrogantly. I mean it from a healthy perspective and life experience. You can let someone into your life too soon, only to be hurt, discarded, and left behind, as I was. Your pillar people need to be there to support you and accept you with your fragility, without hesitation. These are loving, caring people who will gladly accompany you on your heart journey of transformation. Mine helped me feel confident and free with my imperfect self, which helped me to accept my fragility and vulnerabilities. You are not alone and you don't have to do this alone. If you are wondering who has the honor of being your pillar people, here are some words to describe them: they help raise you up, inspire you, encourage and support you, and are not self-absorbed. They care for and love you while moving you in healthy ways.

Who are your pillar people and what role can they play in your continued recovery? Accept the blessing of having people help you with your transition home and through your recovery. This combination of special souls will create stronger bonds with you and amongst themselves. Maybe an old bond comes front and center again in our life. Maybe a weak bond ends up eventually breaking off. Whatever happens, it's OK and we will be OK.

PLACE & SPACE

First and foremost, you and your number one pillar person need to decide together where you are going to go to recover and how the space will be carved out for *only* you: your place and space. Give it some thought while in the hospital and discuss it with your pillars as a great start to your heart journey. You might be wondering why this is deserving of your attention right now, when all else seems to be spinning around you. It is extremely important because the place and the space you recover in will be what's going to feed you mentally, emotionally, and physically for a while. You want to be where you can heal in positive ways, surrounded by loving support.

Here are some words to describe the *place* that would be most suitable for you to recover in and the *space* you will most benefit from: a cozy, lovely room or a full home, yours, a friend's, or family member's, that will be your refuge or sanctuary, a peaceful room that is a clean space, quiet when needed for sleep, windows for sunshine and fresh air, close to a bathroom. The space where you recover needs to be free of as much stress as possible: No yelling, fighting, abusive types of behaviors, or continuous loud noises like home repairs or outdoor construction. The space which you call your room needs to be only for you and includes the things that you need for your comfort. Being with your furry friends is also a huge plus for boosting recovery factor.

Stuff to include in the place and space might be: journals for writing or a pad of paper for lists and notes, books to read, something for music, your phone and charger, a PC, access to a television if it is important to you, and so on. Having the place and the space to come home to will not only boost your morale, but will make you feel relaxed, comfortable, and ready to recover. Make a conscious choice for yourself and give yourself this gift. This is one of many actions you will take on your healing journey that provides you with a returning sense of control and lessens fear. You are alive. You did survive. Now we move on to thrive.

PEOPLE

Once you arrive home, take time to make a list of your support network, where you build and have the collaborative relationships to help you heal. By taking this action, you will see on paper that you will not be alone. You will have a village of supportive humans helping to care for you because you are blessed. This will include anyone that are friends or family members, boy/ girlfriend or partner that steps up to the plate unabashedly to be part of your care team. In addition, they can help you become educated about your circumstances, in order to make the changes you need to. All of this creates a semblance of control coming back into your life. New habits will become ingrained into your daily schedule by your support network.

Your support people will have visits with you, take walks, go grocery shopping, cuddle with or make meals for you. Your support network includes anyone within the sphere of medical support: your cardiologist, primary doctor, rehab physiologists, nurses, physician assistants, and even your phlebotomist. When you need to, you can reach out to them or a pillar peep can on your behalf. Connecting with them on as a needed basis will prove to be very beneficial. Some of the folks that I got to know on a first name basis and have since become good friends of mine are my phlebotomist, Eric and my pharmacist, Natalie. They are such cool, helpful people!

I also made new friends in my cardiac rehab class that became part of my support network. "I have been where you are and I know how you feel," became a powerful and comforting statement to hear. Connection and bonding are soothing as you go through your lifestyle changes. Every one of your network connections will provide different insights, knowledge, shared experiences and valuable recommendations from their unique life experiences. There is a plethora of help out there, in person through daily human interactions, as well as online. Heart attack survivor support groups are available as an amazing resource as well. Reading survivor blogs is very inspiring and helpful. Check this out online to find survivor groups that meet your needs.

At this point, it becomes important to start being mindful about letting go of some control, by allowing others to help take care of you. It may be a struggle at first, especially if you are a Type A person. My dear friend Wayne used to say, after surviving his second heart attack coupled with bypass surgery, "I realized that my biggest struggle was my triple-A personality. From the time I left the hospital and through my whole recovery period, I had to learn to become mindful of this triple-A mindset. It was my worst enemy." Wayne had a primary pillar person that was also his caregiver and his girlfriend all wrapped up in one. He found his salvation by recovering in his safe places: his condo, the yoga studio, and out for his meditative walks in nature. He started losing weight, eating better, and enjoying less stressful activities. In Wayne's wonderful words, the three most successful things he did to recover and heal were to change his playground, his playmates, and his playthings. Voilà!

Another nurse friend of mine was recovering from a heart event at the same time I was. She shared with me that she hated the feeling of not being in control as she placed her life in the hands of her fellow medical staff. But by taking control and setting up her place and space, once she got out of the hospital and home in her sanctuary, she started to feel relief from the sense that some control was seeping back into her life. She journaled a lot and began to understand that fear and feeling helpless is normal. Her husband became her primary pillar person and she welcomed the support of family and friends, even including her young kids, by giving them daily tasks to help out. She did not cope on her own. Please do not cope on your own. There is no benefit or need to. Isolation is not your friend. Let your support network bless you with help so you can concentrate on carving out your new life.

It will take some time to build this network along with new, daily routines in your place. But soon enough, you will look around and realize that you have created a social support system that will encourage you to adhere to your treatments, meds, and lifestyle changes. There will be a dance that starts to emerge from the coming together of moving parts of people and things. Intense periods of emotions and feelings will come about as you establish the new ground that is forming under you. Think of yourself as a seed. A seed needs attention, warmth, nutrition, and hydration in order to grow and burst out of the lonely, dark ground in which it was trapped. You are a seed that needs to turn fully inward, and then upon soaking up all that is required for you to grow, you burst out of the ground with passion, excitement, and momentum to become a sapling. This is exactly what you are doing during this recovery time.

BLIND SPOTS

You may be worried about or wondering about the demanding set of obligations you left behind, like your job and the pile of work stacking up. The response to that is simple: no grand gestures. There will be no grand gestures, as my sister frequently says. There is nothing more important than your health. If you don't recover and regain your health, you have nothing, especially that job. So, no grand gestures. There are ways and choices that can be made to position your health and self-care as the number one priority.

A blind spot is something that causes a person's view to be obstructed. As you endure this experience of a heart ailment, your vision will surely have blind spots, things that you don't really see or don't accept as realities. Ask your pillar people to point out if you are making unhealthy decisions about your job. They love and truly care about you, have your best interest at heart, and remain instrumental to your healing. Clarity around choices, patterns, and behaviors can be identified by them if you ask. Share this stuff with your Pillar People. Trust and rely on them for help making difficult decisions. They will be instrumental in helping you identify crucial blind spots, like your job and how to handle it.

Discovering blind spots related to your heart attack can be an eye-opening process and a necessity to healthy well-being. The key here is becoming aware of them as a crucial step in order to face them, recover, and heal. Here are some example blind spots brought to my attention by my pillar kids: (1) needing more consistent daily eating habits, (2) getting cardio exercise more than a couple of times a week, (3) dumping the heavy load of my very stressful job, and (4) being honest with myself about how some people in my life that I thought were pillar people were really unhealthy for me.

Who within your support group can help you identify your blind spots? What are their particular areas of expertise or life experience that they can share with you to address your blind spots? My soul-sole daughter Courtney is a certified nutritionist. She was so helpful on the changes I needed to make with my diet and exercise. My sun-son Dalton talked to me about less tangible blind spots, some that I had been struggling with for years. One of these was coming to terms with the roles that men played in my life. This included my father's past role, brother, romantic partners, male work colleagues, and even my son himself. We talked about what roles they played and play, and identified what roles I needed the men in my life to fulfill, especially now with my recovery. I made much progress in this area.

For a long while, I didn't see the full picture around these blind spots. Hence, the word "blind." But after deep and lengthy conversations with my pillar kids about these key topics, I was able to identify them, reframe, and redefine their purposes and take healthier actions and attitudes toward them. This was a form of self-love, a step in the right direction for me to actively put myself first, before my roles as a mother, sister, daughter, romantic partner, professional, friend, or neighbor.

The blind spotting process was a dynamic time for me, an experience that became natural and free-flowing. It is very empowering. It doesn't matter how your blind spots materialize. Discovering and identifying them must occur first before the second steps can start: doing the work to redefine them in order to move forward. The people in your support network will help you with this. They were not brought into your life by accident. You were meant to cross and share life's path together. If you have kids, their spirits have also come to you on earth for a reason. Every person in your life is here for the purpose to either help change your life or for you to change theirs. Be grateful for the paths that have crossed and are crossing. Be grateful for the connections new and old. Be excited about the new growth you will take with your pillars and support network. The best of your heart journey is yet to come.

GETTING ORGANIZED

In parallel with identifying pillar people and creating a support network, this is also the time to get organized. What will be your daily movements, rituals, routines, and disciplined duties needing to be attended to? How can your pillar people help you with these matters once you are home? When my kids read this section, they will laugh because I have been in a perpetual state of getting organized! It fundamentally reduces being overwhelmed, saving energy and relieving stress. Most importantly, you gain a sense of control. For me, getting organized after my heart attack was challenging because I couldn't muster up the energy and didn't have a system to refer to. For you, having access to the organization process from this book will allow your energy, time, and mental space to be dedicated to healing as you walk through this system.

First, when you get home, you will immediately be thankful that you purposefully gave time to selecting where you were going to heal and how the space would be prepared. Find a folder and put all your valuable papers and material documents in: catheterization results, prescription slips, doctor reports, pamphlets from the hospital, discharge papers, et cetera. Having them in one place means using up less energy to access them when you need them. As time goes by, you will pitch some and re-arrange others, but having them in one place is for your ease, as well as for your support people. If you live in a smart home, and have Google Home, Amazon's Alexa or Apple's Siri as a digital smart home voice assistant, this is where you will really get your money's worth. These artificial intelligence ecosystems will be able to assist you tremendously with your to-do lists, tasks, listening to music, et cetera. Give some serious consideration and planning to how they can best serve you during your recovery and healing time.

Medications

Find a container to put your prescription medication bottles in as well as any supplement bottles. A basket or Tupperware container works well. Leave it in the same cool place for everyone to have easy access to. It will take some time to remember medication names, when to take them, their dosages, their purpose, and interactions. Keeping up with everything around your meds can be a challenge. Once they are in one place, you or a support person can make a list of them, their dosages, and times to take them. Add your pharmacists' names and phone numbers to this list for easy access. Put the pharmacy info in your phone as well. Then, make several copies of this list: one for you, your wallet, on the fridge, and for your pillar people. Have someone on your support team create your medication schedule. Put reminders in your cell phone and promise to stick to the schedule. Don't take more or less of any of the meds prescribed. If you forget something about them, and you will, write the question down and call your pharmacist. If you are concerned about supplements that you take, like vitamins, write this down to discuss with your pharmacist, the person you will soon become friends with. Take note of when to call in refills. Put this in your phone as a reminder too.

Then, have someone buy a pill organizer for you, preferably one that has multiple compartments – morning, noon, evening, and bedtime – depending how often you will have to take meds. This makes it super easy, as this is a container that you can take around the house, put somewhere that is easy access, or when the time comes, take on trips. It's best to get a container where the compartments are large, easy to open, and snap shut securely.

Don't be surprised if this medication organizing is an emotional event. It was for me – I couldn't even deal with it for the first couple of weeks. My kids had to do it for me. All of it. At age fifty-six, I was a med-virgin. Looking at all of those "disgraceful" pill bottles brought me shame and humiliation because none of this was supposed to happen to me. Was I in a time warp, back in my parent's kitchen on Kingfisher Lane in Clarkston, Michigan, sorting out their pills for them because they were too sick to do it, or maybe in the process of dying? Maybe I was back in time at Hallman's Apothecary on Main Street, with my eight-year-old hand holding my father's hand while he carried out his bag of scripts, always saying to me, "Lisa, make sure you always have medical benefits with your job, honey." That's what it felt like to me. I remember those days like they were yesterday. I also remember telling myself that this would never happen to me, that I would do any and everything to avoid going on any pills. Yet, there I was, flash forward to the present day, watching my kids sorting, compiling, and reading labels. I wept and then retreated back to my safe place, under the covers of my bed with my dog Nahla. As time went by, I would remind myself that I hadn't died. I wasn't going to die from this and I would live for many more years to come. The weeping subsided and I held tight to what my cardiologist said: "You will most likely get to come off several of these meds over time, if all continues to go well." He was right. As time went by, I did come off most of them.

Groceries

After you've put all your papers together and have your

meds in control, it's time to stock your pantry. Get someone to make a list of all the heart-healthy ingredients you will need from a grocery store run. Reference the Heart Healthy Nutrition appendix at the end of the book for a sample grocery list. Have a pillar person rearrange the cupboards and the refrigerator to accommodate the new foods and pitch out the junk and processed items. If you have family members that don't like this approach, have them separate the space to accommodate everyone. The point is to create your own space. Remember and remind your other household members that you already survived a heart attack and now it's time to pull out all the punches to prevent another one by embracing daily heart-healthy nutrition.

Commit to eating much healthier. A nutritionist may have visited you in the hospital, or you will certainly learn from one in your cardiac rehab program. You can also go online to learn a lot. Knock yourself out on eating a heart-healthy diet everyday of your life, one meal at a time. Make a commitment, truly to yourself, to eat well. Create a commitment letter to sign and share it with your support group. A great place to post it is on your fridge. Here is an example to get you started:

"I will move forward, adopting better life-long healthy eating habits for my lifetime. These changes will be very effective in making me healthier and preventing diseases from progressing. I will work to eat a heart-healthy diet, watch my salt intake, and consume fresh fruits and vegetables, along with fish and lean poultry. I will educate myself on the DASH diet and what a full healthy-heart diet is all about, and post it on the fridge for all to see."

Cardiac Rehab

One of the first phone calls to be made will be regarding a cardiac rehab program. Hopefully your cardiologist recommended one to you. They may not have you start right away, with immediate rest being the priority. I started mine a month after my heart attack. If your cardiologist hasn't talked to you about this, call them to gain an understanding around it as well as around the insurance coverage. Cardiac rehab is usually a critical component to recovery. Some people do not want to participate in it because they are afraid of what might happen. Sometimes there is what they call a graduated exercise program. If you got the green light from your doctor, understand all the details that relate to your cardiac rehab program, because you can benefit greatly from the program. It is true that in rehab you will exercise very gently, at your own pace while you are on a heart monitor, with blood pressure checks and medical staff right next to you. What better place to recover and regain confidence in your body than in this safe place?

One Hour On, One Hour Off

With all of these activities going on around you when you get home, you might wonder how to go about your day. First of all, honor whatever restrictions you have. Share those with your support people so you are aligned. Then, you can proceed with your day with a method that served me well. I started off with one hour of normal daily activity, followed up with one hour of rest, usually on the couch or in my favorite reading chair. As the days went by, I felt stronger while adapting to my meds, and my kids suggested that I increase that hour to an hour and a half.

Soon after the first couple of weeks in recovery, I was up to two hours of normal activity and two hours off. It took my scientist kids to come up with this method, but the approach worked, and it gave me a sense of control. A huge shift occurred when I did not need two naps during the day. I knew then that my body was healing and that I was well on my way to being healthier and creating my new life.

With your support network intact and your place with space organized, it is time to 'Unpack Your Crap', the next step in the Heart Healing Process ™. This will provide clarity to you which will help regain your confidence.

STEP 6 — UNPACK YOUR CRAP

"Experience is concrete; it happens to us no matter what. Meaning is malleable; we take with us what we choose to see and choose to dwell on. Dwell on what empowers you. Discard the rest."

— DALTON ROBERT GEORGE, *PH.D., APPLIED ETHICS & POLICY OF BIOTECHNOLOGY, NC STATE*

This chapter is one of my favorites because it's about moving from having a broken heart (literally) to a place where your heart is free (myheartisfree.com) by aligning your mindset with your *heart-set*. By the end of this chapter, you will understand the importance of uncovering life stressors related to the past that most likely contributed to your heart event.

In *Unpack Your Crap*, "crap" equates to the deep-seated issues, patterns, and stressors that have been crammed into your mind and heart containers, creating undue pressures while releasing unhealthy levels of cortisol throughout your body. You will unpack these stressors, one at a time, like emptying a suitcase whose contents you have forgotten. The articles in your suitcase consist of pieces of relationships, work stressors, home experiences, and other difficult matters of the heart, that need reconciliation in order for healing to occur. You will further learn how to unpack your mental crap in exchange for much healthier headspace, learning how stress affects your life negatively. The emotional state of your mind directly feeds your heart. What's lurking in both the shadows of your head and heart is what brings you down. By unpacking your crap, you open up the real estate between your ears, making room for all the new, beautiful beginnings that you will create for your post-heart attack abundant life. Taking care of number one is vital so that you don't fall into number two: Crap!

In this chapter, I will share examples of the life stressors and issues (crap) that occurred leading up to my heart attack, and demonstrate how I unpacked them. My hope is that my examples will resonate and help you to follow the same process to unpack your crap *as they occur* in your life. Learning to unpack a life stressor in real time, as they happen, versus letting them stack up, is so much healthier for our body, mind and spirit.

There is always a lot more content in the life stressor descriptions because this is where you sort through everything, reflect upon it, and then unpack it. Unpacking is where you analyze its value and whether or not it serves you to keep it. It's unpacking it that brings you relief and freedom, because you have addressed it with your Truth, capital T, and follow up action (calls to action).

When I took the time to sit back and really think about what my life had consisted of the year or two prior to my heart attack, I was stunned to realize the trend of negative energy, darkness, heavy events, and stressful experiences that hit me up month after month. Life was not balanced with joy, fun, laughter, or love to tip the scales in my favor. Here is my list of life stressors as examples for you to use as a comparison to the list of your pre-heart attack life stressors you will compile for yourself.

LIFE STRESSOR: FAMILY CRISIS

Shockingly, one of my siblings suffered from and survived the widow-maker's heart attack. This type of heart attack is caused from a one hundred percent blockage of the left anterior descending (LAD) artery. It is also referred to as a CTO: chronic total obstruction. According to the AHA, the survival rate is only twelve percent. This was beyond scary, to have one of my siblings suffer from this shocking event. I chose to take action to help support them and tried to visit as much as possible. On one of my favorite visits, shortly after the event, we went out to feed the ducks. My sibling shared with me that being with the ducks was the most peaceful time for them because the ducks, as do all animals, force a person to be in the present moment. We had a long talk about the importance of being and staying in the present moment because it grounded a person after a crisis situation and was mentally healthy. We also talked about how lucky it was that he had benefited so greatly from the advancements of medicine and technology.

Unpacked

Unpacking (reflection, analysis, thinking about or studying) this kind of life stressor can be emotionally overwhelming, fraught with contemplation about family genetics, coupled with the realities of heart attack disease's role in our family. My first *call to action* was to do the best I could to help them during that crucial time with heartfelt blessings. I remember crying a lot because of the pain they went through with this heart crisis. The detailed recollection of how it all happened was overwhelming.

As I unpacked this shocking event more, another concern developed. Was I doing enough to ensure I was not in any danger? As a result, I had another *call to action*. This widow-maker heart attack triggered me to see my doctors right away and have more tests done to ensure that I was not at risk for a heart attack. This call to action provided me with the reassuring medical reports I needed to not worry about my health.

I also kept thinking back to our duck walk, and for me, knowing how animals do draw you in to live in the present moment, I decided I needed to start living much more in the present moment. This was also a huge takeaway for me. I decided that it was time to get my next rescue dog. It had been six months since I lost my GSP rescue, Casey, at fifteen years old. I had another *call to action* and behold, two months later, my beautiful Nahla was in my life, rescued from a kill shelter in Alabama.

All three of my calls to action were God working through my sibling's heart event to get me moving in better directions. Every day of our lives, we are shown, through other people and their experiences, what we truly need in our lives, if we are open enough to see the messages and callings. If you are living or thinking too much in the past, you will be faced with depression and regret. If you are thinking too much in the future, you will feel overwhelmed and have anxiety. But not when you are living in the moment.

Lastly, I also had to unpack the reality that my sibling may or may not go to cardiac rehab. As much as I was a firm believer in this therapy, many people choose not to go to cardiac rehab. This is their personal business, as I am not privy to all the personal details of any heart attack victim. What I can say is that there is a lot of fear we must face after an event. Fear of having another heart attack if we push ourselves too much. Fear of medical bills if there are challenges with insurance coverage. Fear about losing a job and the challenges around returning to work. The point is to not judge someone who is on their unique heart healing path, for each needs to face and live their own Truth.

LIFE STRESSOR: SUICIDE GRIEF

The year before my heart attack, a very close friend suffered from the traumatic loss of her brother to suicide. This resulted in a very heavy time of shock and grief that lasted the whole year prior to my heart attack. Watching her cope with the worst ordeal of her life was difficult for me and exhausting. We rode the roller coaster ride of emotional ups and downs for over a year together. She became swallowed up by the shadows of her mother's stroke illness, the brother's suicide, spending much time visiting the cemetery, going to many local funerals, and tending to estate demands. We stopped having any fun together and I was walking on eggshells whenever in her presence. I felt so badly for her, having to run the gauntlet between confusion and guilt that haunted her on a daily basis from family suicide, all while trying to care for her sickly and elderly parents. Let's unpack this.

Unpacked

Upon reflection, I realized that I supported her as much as was humanly possible. I also witnessed, as the year passed by, that she continued to get to angrier, more frustrated and exhausted from the result of tragic events that happened in her life. Even though she was prompted to seek help, she did not receive the support she needed in order to heal. As a natural by-product of the suicide experience trauma, simple communication became challenging and the bond that we had crumbled. My call to action was to retreat to give her the space she needed to fully take care of her life on her terms while I reset myself to the demands of my own life. I also felt that as time passed, a darker energy became an all-too-familiar vibe that became worrisome for me to continue absorbing. We eventually went our own ways, as sad and as painful as it was. Life came at her hard that year and she was doing what she needed to do to hang on.

LIFE STRESSOR: DEATH

During the year prior to my heart attack, my elderly godfather's health rapidly declined. He was living in loneliness from missing my aunt the last four years and went from being a very active, talkative man with a strong life force to being bed-ridden in a nursing home. Watching him fade away brought back so many memories of my dad's and my mother's demise. I was triggered a lot and found myself mourning the loss of my parents along with eventually losing him. He was the last relative from my mother's Italian side of ten kids. Losing anyone we love at any time can be very difficult. When it happens during a time in your life when a lot of other stressors are going on, it can feel over-the-top depressing and difficult.

Unpacked

One of the healthiest things to do during times like this

is to see that person as much as you need to and this is what I did. Ask them any questions that you need answered. Do not let them leave this world with you having any regrets about your relationship with them, if possible. That is the takeaway here. I loved this man so much. When I saw him for the last time, the night before his morning passing, he just stared at me while telling me how much he missed me, loved me, and was glad to be going home to heaven to be with my aunt. That was the greatest of gifts. My *call to action* after he passed was to spend as much time I could supporting my friend Robby with his deteriorating parents and helping them out because I knew time was of the essence.

LIFE STRESSOR: JOB STRESS

During the year before my heart attack, my corporate employer had put several of us, including me, on a performance plan that we had to pass with flying colors in order to retain our jobs. They did this every August as a way of "restructuring" the organization. This year, it was my turn. I was put on a performance plan that I flew through with flying colors because I worked my ass off like I always did.

Unpacked

In twenty-eight years of working in the global IT business, this had never happened to me before. I realized that my eating, physical activity, and vacation times were greatly disturbed due to the pressures of excelling through the performance plan. This put undue stress on me physically and emotionally. Job stress is horribly bad for our health, something we all know too well working in our Western world. Be fully aware of the levels of job stress.

Merriam-Webster Collegiate Dictionary, Tenth Edition, defines stress as "a physical, chemical, or emotional factor that causes bodily or mental tension and may be a factor in disease causation." BAM, right there, "disease causation." Having loads of cortisol dumped into your body day after day, in a state of bodily and mental tension, will alter your health and impact any equilibrium in your life. It did mine.

Stress is tension, and I was not getting the relief that I needed because I could not take time off. I was working twelve-hour days, doing three people's jobs, and living with chronic stress from sustained work pressures. This was not the ordinary stressors of daily living but the chronic stress from sustained excessive tension. It was a lengthy process for me to unpack the situation that I was in. A lot of journaling was done, talking with friends and colleagues, as well as thinking about my future and what I wanted. Input from my kids helped a lot, as they were both eagerly encouraging me to leave corporate America behind and telling me how much better my life would be. It was then, through other people, that I actually realized that the hesitancy came from me not knowing what I wanted to do after my IT career.

LIFE STRESSOR: A SICK PET

My beautiful German Shorthair Pointer, senior dog Casey was very ill and needed to be put down, but with everything else going on, I couldn't emotionally handle losing her. It would have put me in the loony bin. I would carry her outside to do her business, cuddle her up in blankets at my feet while I worked, and moved her into my bed to sleep with me at night. She hung in there for me, her eyes never wavering away from where I was. When I got off my performance review from work and felt more secure in my job with much less pressure, she was put to sleep. As a result, from busting through the performance review and putting my dog to sleep, I fell into a lonely, short period of situational depression.

Unpacked

I felt genuinely okay with how I handled my dog's situation, but the daily ongoing stress remained pretty high for many months. I remained loyal and dedicated to ensuring her comfort 24/7. She was there for me and I was there for her. I called in back-up to go with me to help with the process of putting her down. Keeping her by my side for a little while longer was what I needed for my self-protection and healthy well-being.

LIFE STRESSOR: JUDGING BEHAVIOR

An ancillary development that caused a lot of angst the year before my health setback was from the dismissal and negative treatments I received from some people. I am sure this happens to everyone at some point in their lives, when we are around people that we know do not care for us, as evidenced by judging eyes and glares. Our feelings get hurt and it is draining in every way. If it is a repeated dynamic, where we are always uncomfortable around a certain person or having to walk on eggshells, we have to take action to back away and avoid being around them. They are not good for our mental or physical health.

Unpacked

When this life stressor was combined with the other life stressors, it all becomes magnified and overwhelming. I am sure you have experienced situations with people in your life who treat you unfairly, are controlling, and judge you relentlessly. Over time, it takes a toll on you, especially for someone who is a heartfelt person. In retrospect, I needed to be less reactive *inside* about how I was misjudged and ignored, to keep myself more grounded.

A lesson learned for me was to create and honor a call to action: If a person is not even willing to talk to you about your relationship in order to understand where the other is coming from for alignment to occur, there is no point in continuing to try to make a positive connection. It's wasted energy. Walk away.

TOXICITY

When you Unpack Your Crap and reflect on the life stressors prior to your heart event, ask yourself this: What things fed and filled your heart with love, fun, positive connection, cuddling, kissing, laughter, enjoyment, and adventure? If you don't have these from the positivity spectrum, you most likely became drained and filled with the dark energy that wore you down. In retrospect, you can see how you spiraled downward. Looking at your specific life stressors, pre heart attack, helps to realize what stress contributed to it.

When learning about life, looking at the people who are in your life, the roles they play and the relationship you have with them, is of vital importance to heart health. These are folks that you see on a regular basis, those who come and go, and others who float in and out when it is convenient: friends, neighbors, family, romantic partners, past and present, anyone who has access to you. Yes, that is correct: access to you. I want you to write them all down. List out your closest pillar people, support network, people you hang out with, old friends that pop in and out of your life unannounced, and family members who you interact with on the occasional holiday or on a rare weekend.

Basically, you will end up with a list of everyone that gets your attention and time, some more than others and some occasionally. With each person, ask yourself if these words come to mind when you think of them: making you feel like you are walking on eggshells; being angry at you; making you feel inadequate with their sarcasm or minimizing comments; acting like they are right all the time; not accepting responsibility for their negative behaviors toward you; holding grudges; gaslighting; having emotional outbursts toward you or controlling, harsh criticism; not allowing you to express your feelings and when you do, dismissing them; lying to you; difficulty trusting them; one-upping you all the time; humiliating you in private or public; only being available on their terms doing what they want, when and how they want it; or starting confrontations a lot.

If you have anyone in your life with a lot of these characteristics, you need to dig deep to realize that they are not healthy for you and ask yourself why you continue having them in your life. People like this bring you down, feed you bad vibes while you soak up their negative energies. This is toxic to you and your heart. You are absorbing all of this into your organs, muscles, tissues, and this influx of toxic energy will continue to affect your health. Yelling, angry outbursts, disappointed looks, degrading comments about your body, sarcastic injections, or constant picking on you erode your self-esteem. After a while, you won't know who you are anymore, and your heart will ache.

Here are words to describe the opposite, people who will feed your heart and soul with positive juju. Allow them to fully stay present in your life and maximize your time with them: caring, loving, respectful, has your best interest in their forefront, tender with what you have gone through, fun, non-judgmental or controlling, lives from the heart, allows you your freedom and to be an individual, respects your thoughts and feelings, growth oriented, empowering, honors you and your body, doesn't suffocate you, and makes you feel safe and protected when we are with them. These people will want to be with you, sitting in the pew next to you at funerals. Riding in the car beside you. Listening to the frogs' croak in the dead of night with you. Being by your side when you are down. Taking care of you while you are sick or playing basketball with you in the driveway when you are in good health. People in your post heart attack life have to deserve to be in your life now because you are leading it heart first. And there is no better time to make changes like this than in the recalibration step in the next chapter.

STEP 7 – RECALIBRATE

"It doesn't happen all at once," said the Skin Horse. "You become. It takes a long time. That's why it doesn't often happen to people who break easily, or have sharp edges, or who have to be carefully kept. Generally, by the time you are Real, most of your hair has been loved off, and your eyes drop out and you get loose in the joints and very shabby. But these things don't matter at all, because once you are Real you can't be ugly, except to people who don't understand."

— MARGERY WILLIAMS, *THE VELVETEEN RABBIT*

You have gone through six steps so far, and have some light science under your belt now. You've looked at how shame and guilt can be felt and dealt with. You've named your pillar peeps, and are working toward uncovering why and how you had your heart attack. You have even unpacked the major life stressors leading up to the event. What do you do with all of this magical information? I call it magical because it is a magical gateway to your healing. Many mysteries have dissipated that eliminates some of your uneasiness. A specific plan can be created that will move you through your unique healing process. You will recalibrate, taking this knowledge and molding it in positive, healthy ways that will enhance recovery. At the end of the day, it's all the healing journey leading you to live your abundant life.

This step requires that you become an active participant in navigating the recalibration process. You, along with your pillar people, will bear the burden of the work necessary to recalibrate. Anything worth achieving in life requires considerable effort and hard work. Recalibration is exactly that – figuring out how to navigate recovery to live a healthy life. You will be creating new, daily routines with a strong emphasis on putting yourself first. You will double down on self-care, something that may be very new to you. It was for me. I thought my self-care was pretty good, but when I did my inventory, there were major gaps.

I realized that I'd been putting others before me for my entire life. First with my parents, then friends, then boyfriends, husband, work colleagues, my adult siblings during their times of need, and of course, always my kids. With recalibration, you will be discovering a new sense of self-awareness that prioritizes putting yourself first; an inner core of strength and conviction invisible to others; a new way of intentional living; an unbreakable bond where you keep your commitments to yourself; and an acceptance of your updated identity. You are becoming an expert on your body with heartbeats of hope, specializing in your own heart attack survivorship for a long life ahead.

Fostering a solid, deep relationship around recalibration and changing might feel scary at first because you have been most comfortable doing things certain ways for a long time. Fear is a stress response, and you have been through a ton of stress to cause this natural response. Because you have already created a safe environment, you are in a space that allows you to take baby steps. Figure out *your* baby steps that are perfectly comfortable for you. A baby step for you is not equal to a baby step for another heart attack survivor. Push others away who question your baby step definitions, because they don't live in your body.

SLO-MO & DRIP, DRIP, DRIP

During the first month after my heart attack, when I was blessed to be on short-term medical leave, everything I attempted to do or complete was in slow motion. It was my "slo-mo" stage. I had a shipwreck of a body that needed a lot of mending and my kids sensed this. They talked to me about slowing down as much as possible. My sun-son Dalton called it the "drip, drip, drip" pace, a pace he said he went to when he was in a funk. So, I approached everything in drip-drip-drip fashion, listening to my body, feeling my heart rhythms and being mindful of restrictions. This pace allowed for recalibration of my daily routines to occur slowly, becoming intentional and diligent in my choices of people whom I spent time with, places I would venture out to, and things I did.

You may wonder if this approach is too limiting, too conservative. The answer is: most definitely not. It is right where you need to be in the short term, anywhere from two weeks to three months before fully returning to normal activities. Hopefully your doctor discussed your specific limitations while working through full recovery. A full recovery is when you are back to "normal," or at least this is how your medical team will describe it. When you hear them saying this, you may think like I did, is it possible to go back to "normal" when you are no longer the same person anymore? I offer this up to you instead: it is not "back to normal" you strive for. It is a state of "becoming," until you reach a new normal.

This new normal will be created by recalibrating your life, making changes that encompass healthier habits, such as daily exercise, eating nutritional meals, greatly reducing stress, and sharing your space with loving, supportive people. Say "I can" and "I believe" to dismiss any untruths about your potential. Be patient and persistent with your approaches. Write them down, being specific on what it is that you will be doing differently and what your goals are. It took you a long time to get to the place in your life where you had this heart attack (years). Then think about how you deserve the necessary time and beliefs in yourself to make the critical changes to prevent and avoid another one.

In addition to slo-mo and drip, drip, drip, another common mantra for me during the recalibration phase was, "Sorry, I'm not about it." This was my response to expectations from others when pressured to bounce back faster than I was ready to. I also got annoyed with people asking me, "You're alright now, right? Everything's okay now, right?" as if it was my responsibility to make others feel okay about what happened and my condition. No, I wasn't alright yet. No, I needed more time. No, I am not going to deny the trauma I experienced and don't expect me to because I fell hard in life this time, hitting rock bottom and breaking into a million pieces, and now I'm trying to figure out which pieces are missing and which ones are still intact.

My first outing during recalibration was with my BFF-sister of thirty years, Geri. She was so sweet, picking me up at a convenient time and selecting an Italian restaurant (because I am Italian) that was small, cozy, quiet, and just lovely. It brought a shine to my heart because she always makes me feel loved and supported. I will never forget that dinner because it was really about me trying out my sea legs, doing some sanity checks with the outer world, and practicing trusting my body again. I recalibrated myself all through that dinner, adjusting expectations like being mindful of the wine bottle at the table because I was on meds. It was one of my first mindful recalibration exercises, and who better to have done this with than my BFF-sister?

STACKABLE MOMENTS

My second outing was much different. It was to a Crosby, Stills, Nash, and Young local cover band concert. I don't know why I agreed to go. Looking back, I wasn't respecting my newfound boundaries, but quickly reminded myself that they weren't fully defined yet. I fell into my lifelong habit of pleasing others instead of putting my needs first. Everything was normal for a cover band experience, except for me. I did not feel normal and I did not have my new normal created yet. There was dancing, drinking, fans going out to the parking lot to get high, very loud volume, and a shoulder-to-shoulder packed bar atmosphere (this was right before the pandemic). Everyone was dancing while I sat on a bench in the back, against a wall, twirling around my nitro pill necklace, holding onto it for dear life in case I had an angina attack in public. Needless to say, I was having a lot of mental anxiety that night. It was too soon to fly the coop and very overwhelming. Live and learn, I thought. At least I dipped my toes into the waters of life.

That evening was what I refer to as a gifted "stacked" experience, or "stackable moments," a phrase I made up some time ago to comfort myself. These are times in life that repeat themselves, come one after another, and you stack them in your mind until you see the trend or the pattern. They can even be with different people at different times of your life, but it's the mirrored meaning of the experiences that makes them stackable, with so much to be learned from them. I had been having a lot of stackable moments during my recovery, and this time was one of them.

You too will have revelations, with laser-focused clarity, around how your life is changing by the day, the hour, and by the minute during recalibration. You will learn to take your time, staying down and out for a while. Don't push yourself. Don't feel pressured by others to have to act "alright." You'll get up and out when you're ready to, when you are stronger, when you know who you are again. Spend your quiet evenings at home, tending to and protecting your heart.

When I was at that concert, I wasn't under the influence of anything to avoid interactions with my short-term meds, but more importantly because I had gained new respect for my body. My son Dalton often expressed that if I found myself having to get a real buzz on before participating in an experience, I needed to ask myself if the situation was truly worth my time. Getting high to get by was not in my playbook, nor was soaking my liver. Instead, I needed to continue formulating the upgraded version of my authentic self.

BELIEVE IN YOURSELF

You will slowly start to believe in yourself again. Attaining this attitude is much easier said than done, especially when you are just coming out of the chaos around the heart attack, procedures, treatments, and hospitalization. You have had a lot thrown at you in a compacted time period and need to process it. By now, you have learned what your prognosis and diagnosis are, and as a result, you many have a mixture of depression, anger, fear, and feeling overwhelmed. You will believe in yourself once you get past the upside-down craziness. You will stumble and fall along the way, but you will get back up and start over. Through this trial-and-error period of recalibration, you are working through feelings, building up confidence, and redefining yourself.

BRAIN GROWTH

During my Whole Life Healing Wellness coaching program, we studied neuroscience, epigenetics, neuroplasticity, and how to heal your brain. I've been able to apply a lot that I learned to my post-heart attack healing process. For instance, our brains primarily operate from established patterns and they default to familiarity, so practicing your recalibrated ways a little at a time and with regularity is important. New ways become naturally familiar to a brain over time. During recovery, there are myriad behavioral changes that can be recalibrated to healthier ways relating to alcohol, caffeine, fats, fiber, cardio workouts, hydrations, supplements, and meds. The longer you have stayed with something, the more deeply it feels familiar to your brain and your body. Remember, your brain wants things to be familiar and will naturally fall into doing things the familiar way, so incorporate changes into your routines with consistency and purpose. When you enter an uncomfortable space, your brain will want to push you back to the familiar. When this happens, literally say to yourself, "No, brain. I *am* going to do this the new way and you will become comfortable with it in due time," and push through.

Making healthy changes to improve your lifestyle directly improves your risk factors, all while your brain creates new pathways to accommodate the changes. Our human brains desire to be growth-oriented, but we make our brains be fixed because we do things the same way all the time. Now that your brain has been experiencing growth, it is happier, prolific, and full of passion, and you are on the brink of your awakening! You are successfully increasing your mental and physical health, which is evidenced through increased endurance, getting stronger, and having more energy and mental clarity. Remember and repeat what works for you until the healthy changes become innate.

Many of us, like myself, grew up with the belief that we are born with a finite amount of brain cells (neurons), that our cells die as we age, and can never be replaced if they are damaged. Newsflash! Scientists today have evidence proving the opposite. According to Queensland Brain Institute, University of Queensland, there is the process of neurogenesis: the creation of new brain neurons. Our brains have the capability to regenerate. Also, with neuroplasticity, referred to as brain plasticity, the brain has the ability to change and grow new connections when we learn new things. The areas of our brain associated with emotions and memories, such as the pre-frontal cortex, the amygdala, and the hippocampus are not hard-wired, they are "plastic," as in neuroplasticity. I highly recommend doing your own research in these areas. It is amazing.

With the changes that you make through the recalibration step, new connections are being formed in your brain. As a result, you will feel more fulfilled, as you become unstuck from the old, unhealthy ways and empowered in the new. Research suggests that each of us constructs emotions from a variety of sources: feelings, relationships, reactions to the environment, experiences, learning, culture, and upbringing. Our brain is lazy, so when it can, it wires thoughts, emotions, or behaviors into circuits that become automated. These automated thoughts, feelings, or behaviors become our ingrained habits, which allows the brain to work on autopilot. During the course of a day, hundreds of habits (automated chunks of our thoughts, feelings, or behaviors) 'boot up' in our brain as we go 'online'. For more discovery on this, a great book to read is *The Brain That Changes Itself: Stories of Personal Triumph from the Frontiers of Brain Science* by Norman Doidge, M.D.

Moving away from a comfort zone, coupled with a fixed mindset, may be a most challenging task. Once you are made aware of having a fixed mindset around some aspects of your life, learning about them and embracing a growth mindset instead will bring a post-heart attack life full of passion, fun, and enjoyment! This is also the place where you will be tuned in to your heart and able to hear and follow its calls.

FIXED VERSUS GROWTH MINDSET

When you have a fixed mindset, your life is boxed in by confining words and phrases like: unchanging; little growth; avoids challenges; gives up easily; expects things to be easy to cope with; ignores useful feedback; and turns down help and support because it highlights defects.

At the opposite end of the spectrum is having a growth mindset, which encompasses the following: understanding that you can change; life is what you make it; creating better situations for yourself; embracing challenges even though the path to the end may be murky; persisting for a long time to achieve your goals and being willing to learn new skill sets in order to achieve them; requesting and embracing critical feedback for personal growth; stretching yourself with belief and conviction; and will using any means, like therapy, experts, mentors, coaches, classes, and nutritionists in order to move forward in life.

With a growth mindset, you can accomplish anything, even reversing heart disease. The latest research says that heart disease can be reversed, and the best way is through attitude, mindset, and lifestyle changes to reduce your specific heart attack risks. Dr. Dean Ornish, the creator of *Ornish Lifestyle Medicine* program, more recently developed the "UnDo It!" program to aid in reversing heart disease. It is a lifestyle medicine program that combines positive thinking, stress reduction, nutrition, exercise, and support. I recommend that you investigate this if you are interested in reversing heart disease. Some key aspects of his program include: losing unhealthy weight, lowering unhealthy cholesterol and blood pressure, cleaning out arteries through nutrition therapy, regular exercise, and becoming your best person yet. In order to do this, you must have a positive growth mindset and push fear aside.

While going through recalibrating your life, one baby step at a time, you will find many silver linings that fill your heart with goodness. One for me was when I got off my sleep meds. I didn't even realize that I had started to take a pill when I had trouble going to sleep, forming a very unhealthy habit. It was a great feeling of accomplishment for me to stop cold turkey while in the hospital for a week. The more silver linings I experienced, the more empowered I felt and the hungrier I became for more.

GETTING SHIT DONE

By week two of recovery at home, it was important for me to complete some form of pre-heart attack normal daily tasks. On those days, I called them "getting some shit done" days. It didn't matter what it was, but getting some shit done meant a lot to me. Sometimes it was little things, like lying on the couch and organizing my greeting cards, playing backgammon with my bestie, or organizing my vast collection of tea bags while throwing some laundry in. It did not matter what it was, but it had to be something. With each passing day, I got a lot more stuff done than the day before. These micro accomplishments will motivate and stimulate you. Every day going forward, you will notice your stamina increasing, your energy returning, and your light shining stronger.

During this time of recalibration, you have to be the leader for yourself. Stepping up can be difficult when you are not feeling well and are tired. I experienced an overwhelming amount of exhaustion the first few weeks, both physically and mentally. Getting myself out of bed on dark, gray Michigan mornings, coupled with the single-digit cold temperatures, added to my exhaustion. I also thought that my new meds were contributing to this mood hangover. These were "funk" periods, as my sun-son calls them.

During funk times, there were many things I did to help myself. I would consciously work on having quality thoughts about myself and you can too. Feed your head, brain, heart, and soul with positive, high-quality thoughts. Use your mind to serve yourself positively, even if you are lying on the couch in the same jammies you had on yesterday. Be your own self-coach, fostering a new relationship by shifting from living a pre-heart attack life to another kind of life. Remember that your brain can handle it and change. Journal about it. Write lists of the things you want to do for your health and make a vision. Create the vision you have for yourself through recovery and healing.

Through the recalibration steps, you will gain momentum that gets stronger by the day, to help you to focus on the most important things. Here is a list I created of those most important things I call the "Heart Attack Survivor Rights". It's a powerful, on-target list, that helps you get to the core of the what are your new priorities.

You have the right to:

1. Put yourself and your heart first.
2. Spend as much time in your heart safe space or spaces, the places that are a sanctuary, a refuge from the world, and that feed your spirit.
3. Allow yourself to experience the full spectrum of emotions you are feeling. Be with them.
4. Not care at all about what other people are doing, saying about you, or not doing or saying about you. Be obsessed with doing your own healthy thing.
5. Understand, in the fullest of details, what happened to you, why, and what can be done about it.
6. Decide who you want to spend your precious time with, as well as remove those who don't provide you loving support or don't have your best interest in the forefront, *always*.
7. Hold back on socializing, invitations, and holiday fanfare as needed.
8. Set new boundaries that not only protect you but help you to grow and discover new things.
9. Make the changes in your life that are required in order to recover, heal, and get strong again.

10. Give yourself permission to accept what has happened, to forgive yourself for what brings you shame, and to let go of blame so that you can restore your heart.

With these ten Heart Attack Survivor Rights, you will be able to keep the mindful connection to your heart strong, make daily decisions more easily and stay strong in your conviction to your healing. In the next chapter, your learnings and understanding about your heart connections will expand even more.

STEP 8 – HEART CONNECTIONS

"The best and most beautiful things in the world cannot be seen or even touched, they must be felt with the heart."

— HELEN KELLER

Now that you have traveled through the many steps of acknowledgment, recovery, and healing, your body, mind, and spirit will shift to a more esoteric level of relating to your heart attack experience during the Heart Healing Process. You reach a point where you realize how eternally connected you are to your heart. It feeds your life force while in this world, then fuels your spirit when passing to the next. What is life force? It is the power within all of us that propels us through our journey on this earth. We each have our own, unique life force within us, and your heart is the connecting life force to the spirit world, your inner world, and to all your fellow humans on this earth. Connection is something that we innately crave as humans, a critical yearning that needs to be filled, and an ingredient for your healing. Being connected to others through our life force also teaches us how to be connected to our own self and Source (God, Higher Power, Prophet, Buddha, et cetera). Your heart is no longer enslaved to the brokenness it had or the damage that was done. Instead, your heart is free and cries out for love and acceptance and for precious connection to grow.

Think of how in sync you are now with your heart, and cherish it at a much deeper level than you did before. It is a living, vital entity within you that is real, tangible, and beautiful, and does nothing but serve you 24/7. At the heart of the matter, this miraculous organ was there for you, working in a damaged capacity to keep you alive, for you to survive your event. Your heart did not abandon you and this is not the time for you to abandon it just because you may be feeling a bit better. Embrace the fact that you and your heart are one entity and without each other, you are nothing. Continue to work on having so much gratitude for that beautiful, beating cardiac muscle that it spills over into your everyday life.

During this awakened phase, you may feel like you are living on borrowed time because you have learned the extent of the damage. Every day has become a miraculous gift, that's how I felt. You love every raindrop that falls, every smile you see, and every tail that wags. Having this awakening is a beautiful experience. Even now, more than a year later, I still wake up each morning, touching both feet to the floor, and say, "Thank you, God, for letting me wake up again today." My dog Nahla stares at me, waiting for my eyes to open, and then jumps to the ground by my feet, knowing that it's time for us to start our day together.

Have you heard this before: "You only have to die once to really learn how to live?" It's so true. Because of your miraculous experience, even on your worst days you innately carry a torch inside, with that magical sensation underneath that everything really is OK at the core and that you are indeed special. *And. You. Are.* Live with this delicately threaded connection, its magical feeling, and your gift of being able to continue with life.

You may have felt helpless at the beginning of your recovery. I did. I needed help with almost everything because I was so exhausted, fighting depression, and had bitterness to contend with. I was able to persevere though because of my heart connection to my amazing kids. Their love sustained me, lifted me up, and helped me. It also helped that they did the grocery shopping, prescription pick-ups, and cooking, which helped me to be on my way to feeling whole again. During this time, I also thought about how some important tasks needed critical attention, like getting my papers in order. It needed to be done. After all, a person could die at any moment and that seemed all too real to me now. The kids and I tackled it together. If you do not have your important papers in order – like a will, health advocate designee, or power of attorney – add this to your to-do list. Get it done with radical attention and acceptance, so you don't have it weighing on your mind.

Reflecting a lot about the mind-heart connection also made me remember this young woman from my hospital floor. She had had a heart transplant a couple of months before I'd met her. After being in the ICU, she continued her recovery on the cardiac wing. When I walked the halls, I'd see her – moving slowly, walking with amazing posture, head held high, talking to people about how she had someone else's heart beating inside her chest and couldn't believe it; someone else had died and because of that, she got to live. She didn't know whose heart it was, what age they were or how they died, but she said that for the first time since being born with CHD (Congenital

Heart Disease), she felt connected to her heart and its energy. She also felt, for the first time, that the stigma associated with CHD was starting to fade and organ donations were on the rise. That was one of the most awe-inspiring heart connection moments I have ever experienced.

HEALING CONNECTION

With this amazing connection, we need to continue focusing on healing in order to arrive at our optimal state of health. By this point in the healing process, you are feeling better, even if it is just a little bit. My cardiologist told me that when heart attack patients start to feel better, they sometimes stop taking their medications, return to unhealthy habits, or ignore restrictions. Please be aware that even though you may be starting to feel better now, you need to continue to be focused on healing, as well as continuing to follow doctor's orders like taking meds.

How does healing happen? What is healing? Healing is your mind and body recovering from injury, in your case, your injured heart. Healing occurs to recover to a healthy state. Parts of you have been unhealthy for a while, including some other systems or body functions, causing disharmony and being out of balance. It's a domino effect. Healing from too much stress, trauma, or tension to your body is necessary. When you heal, you feel relief, tension dissipates, and you start to feel in balance and in a state of equilibrium.

What are some specific ways that you can continue healing yourself? Here are some examples:

1. *Physical methods:* medicines, cardiac rehab, supplements, herbal teas, massage, homeopathic remedies, sitting in the sun, acupuncture, listening to oceans waves, whole-

some and nutritious organic foods, essential oils with a diffuser, or getting a facial.

2. *Emotional methods:* food therapy as a formidable pillar, holding hands, long hugs, other forms of affection, lovemaking, playing music to listen to or actually playing an instrument, laughter, or kissing or cuddling with your cat or your dog. The power of touch releases all sorts of healing hormones, and your responses to loving touch will result in positive emotional energies and mental stimulation.

3. *Mental methods:* food therapy, seeing a therapist, cognitive therapy, meditation, talking with friends, watching a movie, listening to a podcast, hiring a healing life coach, or taking a long walk in the woods to be with nature.

4. *Spiritual methods:* faith, singing in your choir, your religion, church, prayer, pilgrimages, reading the Bible, or through your unique way of praying, you can ask your Higher Power, God, or your Sustainer to send you healing energy as well.

5. *Intention:* a key to healing. There must be intention, both mentally and physically.

Our bodies are miracles with teeny tiny universes and microscopic galaxy systems throughout. Our body has a relentless ability to heal, an innate desire to be healthy and to heal damaged parts and pieces. Our body wants to get back to its state of balance and a state of wellness. Stress and tension can impact this process negatively, so if you are keeping to yourself, in a healing bubble like a hibernating bear in her cave during winter, more power to you! You are intentionally seeking a state of healing for yourself.

During your continued healing time, you may have some serious, stressful emotional experiences that lead to setbacks with your healing process being disturbed. For me, there were some heavy hitters of stressful times. The 2020 pandemic hit Michigan horribly in March 2020, which struck right when I was supposed to start my phase three cardiac rehab maintenance program. The isolation was tolerable but very stressful, and my safe exercise came to a jolting stop. (I did have enough toilet paper though!) There were months of enforced lockdown with an impact on my mental health from the prolonged social isolation. I became a bit dispirited and socially disconnected, falling prey to "lockdown fatigue." There was also a very unexpected death of an elderly man that had become a father figure to me, and one of my pillar people left my life and moved on to a different life.

CONNECTION TO WORK

Choosing not to take the proper time to heal compromises having a healthy body and is primarily a common Western attitude. Don't fall into the trap of ending your healing too early. You only have one heart, body, and life to protect. It's shocking to hear how many people jump right back into their "normal" lives less than two weeks after having a heart event. I've heard stories of people who went right back to work three days after a heart attack. Yes, it is true that the treatment for heart attacks has improved greatly with the advancement of angioplasty and stents in combination with clot-busting meds. Not that long ago, a heart attack survivor was on strict bed rest for the first two weeks, whereas now, with uncomplicated heart events, the patient can be up and out of bed within a couple of days, with a doctor-approved plan to return to work in two weeks.

After listening to many survivor testimonials, I learned of several reasons why people choose to jump right back into life, cutting their healing time short. First, there may have been a lack of medical benefits, including short-term medical leave. Second, the survivor was the main breadwinner of the family and there was a lack of other financial resources to support the family. Third, many women voiced that they felt they had no choice. Their primary role was in domestic home care and their heavy responsibilities called them back too soon.

But the most common reason was denial around the heart event itself, as evidenced by their words: "it was nothing, nothing to worry about," or "it wasn't a big deal and never really happened." These were not just flippant answers either, because when we discussed it further, it was obvious that they did not want to face the fact that their heart event was more than just nothing and was deserving of their undivided attention. Many survivors remain stuck in the denial phase of the grieving process and respond by jumping right back into work. Unfortunately, with further follow-up, I ended up learning that many of them also had a second major heart event within a year after the first. I can't help but only presume that *not* taking the proper time to endure some kind of Heart Healing Process™ contributed to a secondary event. It is a very personal decision, but at the same time, it takes time to make the changes necessary to improve habits and reduce risk factors. There is some published research around this subject via many resources, including *Returning to Work after a Heart Attack*, published April 2012 on health.harvard.edu. Being the knowledge advocate I am, I suggest doing your own research in regard to your own circumstances, to make the best decision for yourself about when to return to work. Successful reintegrating back into the workplace requires forward thinking with a strategic plan, at a minimum. Make wise decisions, because your life depends upon it.

According to the European Society of Cardiology (ESC)'s April 11, 2019 Journal, the main things to consider when making the choice around the return to work include:

- Do you feel like you can go back to work? Why or why not?
- Are there psychological reasons preventing you from being able to mentally return to work, like anxiety or depression?
- What are your medical conditions? Do they affect your ability to physically do your job?
- Are you still learning about how your body reacts to your rhythm instability, ischemia, or implemented cardiac device, which adds to your lack of confidence?
- Do you still have comorbidities that you are suffering from, like obesity, smoking, or diabetes, and need more time to address them?

The best and healthiest approach to these types of challenges or concerns is to seek out the support and input that you need to make the best decision from experts and key individuals, including: a therapist, physiotherapist, social worker, counselor, your cardiologist, or possibly a psychologist.

BROKEN HEART CONNECTION

Have you ever heard of the Vena Amoris? It is a Latin term that means "the vein of love." The Vena Amoris was thought to run directly from your left fourth finger (wedding ring finger) to your heart during ancient times. This was believed to be a very special vein by the Egyptians because they thought it formed a direct connection between the heart and your left fourth digit, the 'love finger'. The Egyptians thought this was why most heart attack victims experienced an excruciating pain that radiates down the left arm from their heart, ending at the tip of the fourth finger on the left hand, the exact same path as the Vena Amoris. Egyptians also believed that the left hand fourth digit, the finger where romantic and love rings are worn, represents sexual and emotional commitment. They called it the "heart finger," or the "love finger" and wearing a ring on that finger ignited eternal love. It is also where the pain of angina radiates to, affecting our wholeness: body, mind, and spirit. Going through a romantic breakup also affects our wholeness, with excruciating pains radiating through body, mind, and spirit.

When my friend Sara experienced a breakup with her boyfriend months after her heart attack, I became very concerned for her well-being. There is so much connection between a person's mental/ emotional feelings to their hearts and body. As I feared, her healing process was interrupted by the unhealthy pressures from his break-up with her. When her heart got broken by the man she loved, trusted, and depended upon, she experienced deep pain, suffering, and heartache, literally. She had a healing setback six months after her heart attack, from the painful loss of losing the love of her life, who was also a main pillar person. She was catapulted into a new phase of grieving due to the loss of her boyfriend, on top of still trying to cope with her continued healing from her heart attack, the pandemic, and many other life stressors. One of the worst experiences you can have while you are in your healing phase is a romantic break-up from a deep love. Healing is just as mental as it is physical and during the first year after a heart event, a survivor faces many firsts to get through, like birthdays and holidays. It becomes very stressful if a romantic partner has been lost.

Why exactly is a romantic breakup so difficult? Let's unpack it.

When you are in love with someone, there are powerful hormones at play that drive your passions and ignite your spirit. You feel attractive and at the same time are attracted to your person. There is much pleasure because of the happy neurons in your brain and the chemicals that are oozing all through your body. It's a wonderful feeling (to say the least), and as a result, deep attachment forms while deep bonds are created. Connection is aligned and all these things are continue happening because of the chemical reactions in both of your bodies. Cortisol rises while serotonin lowers. Love becomes a very complex process involving your brain, heart, and body.

When a breakup happens, your bonding connection and passion-filled heart go into overdrive and you chemically start to crave your person back. Yes, chemically – so you literally feel it all over your body. You may indeed feel like your heart is breaking because you are going through withdrawal from all those amazing hormones and chemicals that were being produced for such a long time. Then you enter a phase of hyperarousal because your emotional regulation system is not balanced, your chemicals are way off, and you deeply miss that other person, chemically, bodily, and emotionally. It sucks, but with time, it passes, as it did for Sara. In due time, her heart healed from the breakup, but the most difficult aspect was the setback in having to start a new grieving cycle.

On behalf of our healing and becoming as healthy as possible, we must learn how to fix, or at least how to manage, a broken heart – literally and figuratively. If this is something that you are faced with during your healing journey, please seek the support that you need to help shepherd you through it. Suffering from a broken heart is nothing less than being human and having these passions of the heart. We cannot get through life without ever experiencing a broken heart, nor can we escape its inevitability. Romance, falling in love, and then breaking up results in a broken heart. Going through a divorce can break hearts as your marriage crumbles. Witnessing someone you love deteriorate from Alzheimer's and pass away crushes your heart. A child born with a congenital heart ailment can break a new parent's heart. These inevitabilities will never go away, nor will they be eradicated. We will all experience a broken heart, in some way, shape, and form, at some point in our lives because we are all human. We cannot escape it, literally or figuratively. It strikes the affluent and the non-affluent. It touches the young, the old, black, white, and brown alike around the world, and is as damaging emotionally as it can be physically. The two go hand-in-hand.

"I can't function, think or get out of bed. I have no energy or interest in life right now. I feel so hollow and empty and defeated," Sara used to say to me as she wrestled with the aftermath of her breakup. "I knew this was coming and I know it's for the best, but it hurts so much, my heart is broken," she shared. You could hear and feel the deep sadness and grief in her voice. Time was needed to heal from this loss and to grant clarity, time, support, patience, faith, and love.

What Sara was able to do then was amazing. She was able to get honest about the shadows that she carried within her heart from this breakup: resentment, disappointment, anger, and grief. She started to journal to work through them. As a result, she began to realize how strong she really was, how beautiful and amazing everything about her heart was. She shifted her dark energy into light energy through gratitude. She wrote about how blessed she was with how her heart takes care of her. She went through a phase where she actually talked to her heart, asking how it was feeling that day, resulting in an even deeper connection between her and her heart. She asked, "What actions can I take to love you better?" She learned a lot from what her heart was trying to teach her.

She went on to learn how to pay attention to the wisdom of her heart by apologizing to it when needed and also reading her heart affirmations: I love you, you are beautiful, you give me strength, you allow me to live, thank you, you are enough, I will be your best friend. She began to live her life leading with her heart, and stayed heart-centered as her heart became her new partner. We want to be that person too, who moves beyond new pains and suffering with courage, strength, and fortitude. We need to embrace our inner warrior to help us during these times, just as Sara did. She unknowingly fell in love with her own grateful heart and self, for the first time in her life. From here, she was in a wonderful place in her life that allowed her to continue to grow.

STEP 9 – POST-TRAUMATIC GROWTH

"The challenges we face in life are always lessons that serve our soul's growth."

— MARIANNE WILLIAMSON

You have survived, coped, and are recalibrating! Now it's time for continued growth with a heart that feels more alive than ever! The Heart Healing Process moves you to a place where you can open up space, fill up on gratitude, and be poised for your new normal. If you are not, don't fret. You are most likely needing to rework through a previous step or are still working on a step. Everyone's journey through The Heart Healing Process varies and is experienced differently. You may not travel through the steps in the same order or in the same time frames. Honor where you are.

When you arrive here, 'tis the season to celebrate because you are in PTG: Post-Traumatic Growth. Yes, PTG and it is a real thing: a significant, positive consequence experienced as a result of a personal crisis. It is a psychological change as the result of a traumatic challenge like a heart event. It is not to be mistaken for resilience, which is the ability to *recover* rapidly. PTG is a whole new level of *functioning*, a phase of positive transformation that follows intense adversity. Psychologists Richard Tedeschi, PhD. and Lawrence Calhoun, PhD., from UNC Charlotte, uncovered this psychological trait in the mid-1990s. There are three main pillars to its concept and theory:

1. You have become a much stronger, personal self.
2. You have much deeper and more meaningful relationships in your life now.
3. You are living with an awakened, ignited spirit.

For me, I was blessed with experiencing all of these sensations and feel that I am still lingering in this stage, a year after my heart attack. Some common sentiments of someone experiencing PTG are: I have a deeper appreciation for every moment of my life now; I know that I can handle difficult things and get to the other side; my priorities have shifted a lot in my life; and I discovered that I am much stronger than I ever thought. Maybe you have been finding yourself echoing these sentiments or others of a similar nature!

There is an assessment a person can take, developed by Calhoun and Tedeschi, that determines the actual level of PTG that a person is experiencing. There is a long and short form of the PTG assessment questionnaire you can easily find online. I've included ten example questions from the short form that are used to evaluate a person's level of PTG. The more you say yes to, the stronger your PTG state is.

- I changed my priorities about what is important in life.
- I have a greater appreciation for the value of my own life.
- I can do better things with my life.
- I have a better understanding of spiritual matters.
- I have a greater sense of closeness with others.
- I established a new path(s) for my life.
- I sincerely know better that I can handle difficulties now.
- I have a stronger religious faith or deeper spirituality.
- I discovered that I'm much stronger than I thought I was.
- I learned a great deal about how wonderful people are.

Not everyone reaches PTG at the same time, and the depth of PTG varies. Based on my talks with survivors, the ability to get to this transformative stage seems to be dependent upon the survivor taking enough time to work through what happened to them. The level of trust in their support network is also an indicator for a survivor's ability to get to PTG, again based on my discussions with fellow survivors. There seems to be a strong correlation between having a healthy, successful support group with getting to a stage of PTG. This makes sense because if a survivor has attentive, compassionate support through recovery and healing, they are enabled for growth. For me, the people who provided the best, most loving support were the ones who listened to the most difficult and worst parts of my experience, respected what I went through, learned and gained understanding from it, tolerated my ups and downs, and most importantly, are still with me today for the long haul.

In Post-Traumatic Growth phase, you experience warmer relationships with the people you have deliberately chosen to keep in your life during recalibration. You have a much deeper appreciation for life itself, on a level many others cannot ascertain because they have not had a heart attack. You have done the hard work of inventory, while your sense of personal strength has grown because you have unpacked your life stressors, which allow you to see the possibilities of *becoming:* a perpetual state of being, a continued awakening filled with growth. The PTG phase is backed up by making decisions that are one hundred percent dedicated to the protection of your heart and focused on your continued healing. This will be the highest and most honorable way of living you'll ever make for yourself.

There are so many more healthy aspects to this PTG phase. Here are six of them:

1) You are making healthier decisions about relationships. When I'm working with clients through their inventory stage, by the time they get to PTG, they realize that people in their lives who cause them constant pain and suffering are not worth their valuable, precious time anymore. By making decisions to reduce their time with those people, along with enforcing established boundaries, they realize how *growing past* these people has given them the power to make healthier relationship decisions.

2) You are eating well and have made the connection between moods, feelings, and food. When I keep a food journal, or when my clients do, they become much more positive about healing through food as a sustainable, new behavior during PTG.

3) Your interests are deepening again because of the

increased energy level. Take notice of this daily if possible. Before PTG, you may have felt depleted, without motivation to do even the simplest of things. Now, you may even have twinges of excitement. I had one client who hardly slept through the night or had energy to pursue her interests when she first started her recovery. By the time she was in her third month of working through the Heart Healing Process, she had been sleeping through the night and began a lifelong dream of being a foster mom to kittens.

4) You have a lot more clarity around what you went through and the changes you are making as a result.

5) You've developed disciplines and structure for your soul to grow and expand.

6) You are more grounded than in the early stages of recovery.

What are you or your loved one experiencing in the phase of PTG? How does it feel and what has changed? What do you love about it and hope lasts? If you are not here yet, what do you hope it will feel like?

BECOMING

The most important word that describes the phase of Post-Traumatic Growth is "becoming." Here, I will talk about what becoming is, how you feel while you continue to become, and the behaviors around it. Becoming is a perpetual state, with eyes of energy looking out into the world, a renewed sense of hope coupled with a grateful heart that carries you. Nothing replaces living your best, authentic life, filled with passion and joy. You may think you are not ready, but you are. You have consciously debunked your mind and unblocked your funk. Because of all these things, you know yourself and uncovered your Truth, allowing you to grow while manifesting what you desire. You have been planting seeds for a while, sprinkling them everywhere, watering them, providing sunlight, and keeping the weeds out. Now it's time to watch them sprout and bloom.

This phase of PTG is not scary but freeing, as you move forward with your leveled-up way of living. You are authentically facing the present and what is coming to you. Your strength from healing will allow you to stay in the present moment. Keep practicing, staying in your present moment, and being aware of how your body and mind feels when you are living in the present moment during PTG.

Post-Traumatic Growth is about making the best decisions for you and your heart, with intentional becoming. Keep your eyes looking through the front windshield and not the rearview mirror. You have successfully moved yourself through a kaleidoscope of emotions, thoughts, fears, perspectives, and assumptions. With actions and movement, you pushed your fears aside and now is the time to enjoy the growth from all of that work.

SUSTAINING PTG

How do you sustain the state of PTG? By continuing to ensure your needs are met and living life on your terms, while looking through the "front windshield." Let's walk through seven areas of your life that need to remain top priority to keep healthy and growing:

- *Physical state:* Stay closely connected with what is going on with your body and your heart, in order to maximize your health, maintain vibrancy, and vitality. Ensure that you continue eating a heart-healthy diet, getting the right amount of exercise

and daily movement, while taking any still-required meds and keeping all of your doctor's appointments. Have a bodacious health plan in place to keep your body in great shape.
- *Keeping a finger on the pulse on your emotional state:* Stay in sync with and monitor your emotions through journaling. Take time every day and ask yourself how your emotions are affecting your heart and how they are created from your mind and your brain. If you don't take the time to think about this, you will not be in sync and they can creep up on you. Healthy, positive thoughts and emotions equals a healthy heart. Negative, raging, and angry type emotions = unhealthy heart and arteries. Mindset equals heart-set. Keeping a finger on this pulse will help you to continue to grow and know yourself, as well as reduce life stressor effects.
- *Beliefs:* Continue clearing out old, destructive, negative beliefs that come back to haunt you. These beliefs will try to keep you from reaching your potential and fulfilling your possibilities. Remember that they are old patterns in your brain that need to be pushed out and reframed with positive, uplifting, and encouraging beliefs. Literally, tell yourself to *not* think in ways that are destructive. Give yourself other mantras to say in place of the old, negative head talk.
- *Relationships:* Be intentional with the relationships you have by making and keeping positive ones in your life. The toxic, negative relationships that hurt you need to be kicked to the curb. Maintain and sustain those that feed your soul and spirit, keep you a priority, and have

your best intentions at heart. Most of all, keep the relationships with other humans that cherish and love you to create your "MWE" community: me + we for the long haul.

- *Self-care:* Spend your time doubling down on self-care, healthy habits, and staying connected and bonded while keeping yourself number one. Make sure that most of what you do to yourself is heart-healthy.
- *Work:* Ensure that you are making the best of your work situation and if it is too stressful, get out. Move on to something that is sustainable and will not put stress on your heart.
- *Spirit and soul:* These need to be fed regularly. Bring joy, love, kindness, prayer, or acts of charity to the forefront. Keep what is needed to feed your spirit and your soul in abundance.
- *Brain reserves*: Keep these in place as much as possible. What are they? Love. Touch. Sleep. Energy. Patience. Nutritious foods. Hydration. Keep your brain reserves high for your continued protection and progression.

You are still recovering and healing, with those best-kept secrets of feeling embarrassment, shame, and guilt right after your heart attack far behind you. You have regained your confidence and restored your control and power by following the steps of figuring out the why and the how behind your event; completing your inventory while painstakingly unpacking your crap; and recalibrating; and the heavy pain and loneliness are no longer growing or intensifying. Best of all, you no longer hide your story, and this was a major turning point in your recovery. All of this allows you to be much more mentally healthy.

Remain strong and easily set your ego aside when needed. You have faced your test results, numbers, genetic and family histories, and no longer run from the past. Instead, you are ready to be propelled into your new future, where the embers of your new life have started glowing. You have worked hard to get through these steps as your roadmap and now you are more than ready to receive the benefits. You have freed up so much of your energy and time that was being taken up by worry, fear, concerns, anxiety, and unhealthy relationships; that now you put your time, energy, and focus on yourself and your sacred heart. You have taken back control and you are your own hero. It's time for you to feed those embers, let them grow and roar into a beautiful flame. Grab your commitment to yourself and the powerful light of hope to continue to change things, make new discoveries, and carve out new paths. You have been washed over with a new level of self-love, respect, and moxie. Welcome to the land of PTG!

CREATING SPACE

What is truly possible now that we've reached the growth stage? What opportunities will present themselves and how does what we went through impact new chapters in life? Remember how you were devastated from your heart event, while fighting exhaustion? This was a necessary phase to endure, a necessary cluster of emotions to work through to get to the other side. For me, once I was at peace with my decision to take a year off and had comfort in knowing that financially I could make it work, the magnificent world of possibilities began to unfold. A space had been created. The space necessary for the world of possibility to appear. Only when we create the space can a new world open. Continue creating space for yourself and your needs.

I also compiled a list in my journal of what I loved, where my passions came from, and what made my light shine. I needed to physically see this list to understand myself again and to help catapult me into this next phase. It had been a long time, since before college, that I had thought in these terms of "just for myself." Journaling became a daily ritual. I also was able to start saying "yes" to opportunities that came my way. Here are some of the manifestations that became real when I got to PTG: enrolling in a healing course to learn about myself; becoming certified in an accredited life wellness coaching program for self-development; joining an all-women, international coffee group; being a judge to a college alma mater competition for their graduate students; and then starting my book writing process. Before I realized it, I was diving back into life with a steady swimmer's stroke.

Ask yourself, what do I want to accomplish in my life now? Here are some starters from my first list for you. At the time, these felt overwhelming and not possible. With time, and working the steps, they became possible and then real: being healthy by keeping up with cardiac work out three to four times a week; eating a heart-healthy diet one meal at a time; taking my couple of meds regularly; keeping all doctor appointments; getting as much rest as I need; spending as much time with my kids as possible; writing a book on my heart attack survivorship; and becoming a heart-healing life coach. These have remained unnegotiable pillars of my new foundation. Keeping them in the forefront of my life remains critical for staying healthy. I am in an exciting phase of continued discovery, a world of possibilities, and a beautiful space where my soul can breathe, expand, and grow.

THE MEANING OF LIFE

Experiencing life in a state of Post-Traumatic Growth is freeing. It is the opposite of having an existential crisis where you ask, "What does life mean?" You know what it means now because you almost lost it. Existential crises are times when you question whether your life has purpose or value, something that most commonly would have happened to you in the early phases of the Heart Healing Process. You know now, like never before, that your life has purpose and value. Having an existential crisis is commonly tied to negative experiences or provoked by a significant event in the person's life, like a psychological trauma or having a major health setback. You experienced a traumatic health setback and faced a shit-ton of introspection about personal mortality. Hence, having your heart attack did provoke and put you in an existential crisis for a while. Now you have emerged, recovered and healing, and entered the stage of PTG. Your new perception of life and your existence is no longer in crisis mode. You have risen above it.

The search for meaning in your life, for meaning of what you just went through has been dutifully addressed in steps of Light Science, Unpack Your Crap, and Recalibrating. You know what it's about. You no longer lack purpose and are not empty. Instead, you have so much to do, to accomplish, and horizons to discover. The experience with your heart attack was a catalyst that catapulted you in new directions. You paid your dues and suffered for a lot of reasons with spiritual anguish, but this force was redirected to help drive you to new ways that bring joy and satisfaction.

My soul-sole spirit daughter Courtney and I had the privilege of spending time in Japan together many years ago. What a glorious experience for both of us. While there, I learned of the Japanese word "ikigai." It means "your most important purpose in your life" or "your reason for living." When we find our ikigai and own it, we will be very content and live a longer, happier, and healthier life. When I began reading about this concept while traveling across that amazing island, I wondered what my ikigai was. I thought and thought about it, made a list of possibilities, but still struggled to come up with the one unique thing that gave me purpose, passion, fulfilled my life mission, or was the reason why I got up in the mornings. The Japanese also believe that your ikigai keeps you happily active and busy through all your years, helps you to grow and expand, and becomes the source of your life energy. I realized that ikigai was very powerful stuff, but couldn't answer it so I let it go.

After I had my cardiac setback, the concept of ikigai came back to me, but it remained difficult to unpack this philosophy when there was so much spinning around. How could I possibly know what my ikigai was? Did I ever know it, like years ago when my life seemed to be so put together and not falling apart? I was in such a different space now, in a new time warp where I was struggling with simply understanding who I was and what I was forced to become. I didn't get to retire from my thirty-year corporate America career, step away from it gracefully, or enlist in a stimulating sabbatical. Instead, I decided to honor my kids' adamant request to take a year off, calling it "resigning" but referring to it as a mid-life gap year. That's right, just like my daughter and all the other Millennials do when they take a year off after high school or undergrad studies, prior to taking the next step like college or a real job. My mid-life gap year was without the flare of the millennial versions: backpacking across Europe or Asia while staying in hostels and meeting all sorts of wonderful people from around the world and eating amazing foods. Instead, it ended up being a year in my sanctuary, writing my book, staying isolated because of the pandemic, and fulfilling God's plan.

I promised my kids I'd take a year off even though I was in an extremely marketable and desired profession. The idea of not working, of not having an income and medical benefits, was strange to me, as I had been working since I was fourteen years old. My kids' sentiments echoed in my mind: "You can fully heal, Mom, emotionally and physically. You can find yourself again, Mom. Take some trips and have some fun, Mom," they said. After a week of gathering all the critical inputs and plunging into my financial details, I announced that I could indeed survive a year off financially. It was with much gratitude and relief that I accepted this blessing of absolute luxury and couldn't wait for this new adventure to start. Within the month, the pandemic set in and writing my book became my amazing, healthy project during isolation.

So, what then is my ikigai? What is the main thing that brings me satisfaction, passion, and joy in life? Was it writing? Reading? My dog? My kids? After much reflection, I realized that my ikigai was not centered on me at all, but instead was centered on the other people in my life, those whom I adored. I lived for the ones I loved and adored and it's through them that I have purpose. I know that sounds cheesy, and I am not holier-than-thou, but I simply don't know how else to say it. What brings me joy and is my higher purpose and calling is "other people," who I can learn from, help with *their* lives, or simply lift them up by spending time with them, like my mom use to say I did.

For the ones I adore in my life, I help in any way I can. Simple ways are the best, like being with them to give them company or for a visit; having a cup of coffee together; hanging out with them as they work on repairs at their parent's house; ironing a suit and giving them a haircut the morning of their dad's funeral; laying on the grass near them while they do outside work; sending gift boxes in the mail; giving goody bags filled with yummy items to help a friend through their day; or providing financial support in times of need, when I can. Getting to the heart of it, nothing is more sacred than simply sharing love, resources, and ultimately time with another human being, a simple yet provocative gesture learned from my dad.

My dedicated ikigai is being in service to others, helping them heal, providing my love, refuge, and nurturing guidance in this very chaotic world. My ultimate ikigai is helping the ones I love to achieve their goals and dreams. That is the higher purpose that makes me want to get out of bed in the mornings with my dog Nahla. Be a rainbow in someone else's clouds (sorry, cheesy), just like the crystal in my bedroom window that spreads rainbow colors all over my walls from the rays of sunshine.

STEP 10 – A YEAR OF GENTLENESS

"When you encounter difficulties and contradictions, do not try to break them, but bend them with gentleness and time."

— SAINT FRANCIS DE SALES

Moving forward with your heart journey and paving the way for the next full year of your post-heart attack life is a monumental place to be in. Hold this thought close for a moment and just breathe, breathe, breathe. Hold it close to your heart and honor this moment in time, where you are going forward, fully alive. It has taken a lot of hard work to travel through this Heart Healing Process™ landing in a healthy place where you can continue to move forward. Congratulations! Now it's time to grab the momentum to move through the next year. You have faced your demons, learned to protect your heart, and implemented well-being strategies with conviction, clarity, and transparency. You are at a pivotal juncture to take your life to the next level, which can be sustained through a year of gentleness. How do you do this? How do you maintain and sustain?

You maintain and sustain your new lifestyle by honoring your healthy changes, mentally, physically, and spiritually. You are the main pillar and master builder. Continue with your healthy steps and actions to ensure that your heart remains a top priority. This chapter is about learning ways that will help you maintain and sustain your healing with positive attitude through your first year, post-heart event.

You have so many tremendous resources at your fingertips to help you continue to move forward. The internet, of course, with all of its 24/7 options for continued research and learning. Keep up with podcasts, TED Talks, YouTube heart topics, and such. You also have yourself, the most important resource. You know exactly what you went through, and that hell is not something to be repeated. This Fact, with a capital "F," is the best piece of evidence to keep you motivated to stay on target with your goals and healthy habits. All the pre-heart attack unhealthy desires will hopefully have disappeared naturally.

You have your support network to be your cheerleader and sounding board. They are there to hold you up during your tough times and tough challenges, especially when life stressors come your way. Keep them accountable for your continued support. They need to know that it takes a full year to really live the new lifestyle that is actively being carved into your every day. It takes a whole year to move through all the seasons, the holidays, and your next birthday, which will feel different for you. And it takes a whole year to work on being gentle with yourself, kind, caring, and filled with self-love practices that are needing to be embraced.

COMMITMENT TO SELF

The most important aspect of this next year is commitments to yourself. For me, I wrote my commitment out. Let's look at it with the purpose of you carving out one for yourself, unique to your own style, and heartfelt needs.

- I will put forth the effort needed to get my heart healthier and to keep my heart healthy.
- I'll slowly re-engage with the rest of the world when my heart is comfortable doing so.
- I will surround myself *only* with those who support my healthy heart recovery and healing; those who have faith in my abilities and are patient with me; those who love and accept me with all my idiosyncrasies; those who accept the new person I am becoming; and those I know and trust are with me for the long haul
- I will continue to grow and really try to learn more about the plasticity of my brain, its connection to my heart, and my heart's ability to recover and heal.
- My heart will continue to be protected by the choices, decisions, and actions that I take.
- Heartfelt celebrations will take place over my triumphs, including a Heartaversary celebration, and on my next birthday: A Hearty Party!
- An attitude of gratitude will be forever a heart mantra of mine. I will create a gratitude journal that I contribute to on a regular basis.
- I am not, in any way, less that I was before. I am more than I ever was before.
- I will do my best to be with people that share

good, positive energy with soft tones and gentle attitudes, open hearts, and a flow of heart-shared love.
- This was an unexpected journey indeed, one that taught me to continue to balance what my head says to what my heart feels and what my gut is telling me. I will continue to balance my head with my heart and my gut.

SLOW-ROLLING IT

During this first year, you may feel like you are moving more slowly than ninety percent of the rest of the world, and that's OK. It was easy for me to stay in this mode because of the pandemic. Regardless, you are where you are and where you need to be. Remember that this is a good thing, it is healthy, and it is a luxury. You will see and experience so much more than when you were living that fast-paced, blinding, and horribly busy life. For me, now that I am not working my corporate exec job anymore, it seems like everything around me is moving in high speed, that the world is on fire and I am watching it from an observation booth. You know what? This is perfectly fine with me. Go at it, other humans, and I shall continue to observe from a distance, safe in my heart-shaped bubble and avoiding a lot of headaches.

When you really drill down to it, your reality exists wherever your mind is. The world around you is going to continue to be poured into your mind's perceptions, regardless of what you are doing. So, continue to guard your mind because what you bring into it, through your lens, becomes your reality. Give your attention to that which you want to become real to you, to that which you allow to take up the precious real estate between your ears.

Said in another way, what's between your ears feeds your heart. Stay mindful of your emotions and feelings, but don't get lost in them. Let go of the ones that don't serve you or your heart and surrender the others that you can't control.

One of my favorite ways to still go through my day when I really need it is via the drip, drip, drip way. What a luxury and a pure joy. You'd think that you are not busy nor active with this approach, but the exact opposite occurs, the difference is your rhythm inside yourself. With drip, drip, drip, you have time to think, reflect, and make proactive choices versus reactive. You have a tone to your day that allows you to breathe and take in the many simple, yet beautiful moments. You are also in a state of mind that allows you to handle waves of emotions. When having waves of emotion, leave them be and let them naturally recede, which they will, like the ebb and flow of the ocean. Don't dwell, ruminate, or obsess over them. Calm all the swirling thoughts and soon you will be back into your rhythm with something creative, joyful, or active.

It is a liberating insight to commit yourself to continue slowing down through your days, finding deeper meanings in the smaller yet profound things, the mundane yet most beautiful. Because of this, you will be filled with more inner and outer energy while enjoying your daily life. Try not to think too much, instead focus on basking in it the day's fullness, comfort, and joy. Having your heart and mind at peace is a gift to be enjoyed: the "present." When you are having a day like this, you will be energetic again, talkative, full of laughter at the silliest of things while allowing the days, weeks, and months to unfold naturally. When this is happening, you will be conscious of it because you'll remember the days or nights when you weren't feeling anywhere near joyful, when you struggled just to get out of bed or off the couch. Train yourself to really feel joy and to remember that many days like this are possible and that they will happen much more often. Notice one key, recurring element associated with this joy: that you are well-rested and you are not dragging around a tired body, heart, or mind. This paired with the key elements of your new, healthy lifestyle are what will continue to propel you forward.

THE COMFORT OF ROUTINE

During your first year, post-heart event, you can add a wonderful friend and comforting supporter into your daily life. Her name is Routine. Routine is extremely reliable, consistent, balanced, wholesome, healthy, and settled – much more than you ever will be. She takes the stress out of daily living by knowing ahead of time what your day will look like. Do you have a regular schedule with specific times for waking up, going to sleep, conscious meal eating, and times for getting some fresh air and exercise? If not, Routine will gladly take care of that for you. Does your day follow a crafted plan that flows easily from one activity to the next, knowing that you will get some relaxation in, some time with friends every Friday night, and alone time for doing what you enjoy? If not, Routine said she'd come to your rescue.

With the many unexpected things that can happen to us on a daily basis, and with the added pressures of the world upon us, having the luxury of routines, rituals, and patterns to follow and depend upon provides security, comfort, and consistent feelings of control. We do not have to be robbed of this peace. Instead, Routine wants to give you this peace. It is through her consistency that our hours, days, and nights are woven together through her power of positive energy. Routine prevents and protects us from all the crazy going on around us. Routine promises that she will give you shelter and refuge from the unexpected bumps and bruises. Once we become conscientious of Routine in our daily lives, we will become pleased to know that there are still opportunities within our routine-shaped days for spontaneity.

The natural web and flow of our days will bring spontaneous happenings, but they are experienced within the safe construct and framework of our daily routine. Instead of our days being puzzles to solve or face every time we get up out of bed, we wake up moving naturally along through our routines with a strong sense of well-being. This can especially be helpful for those of us who must endure long, cloudy, gray winter seasons like myself. There should be no worries or concerns that our routine-filled days will start to feel mechanical or repetitious, because we will quickly notice that our bodies do not feel "off," but that we feel stronger, more confident, and peaceful within our own, natural rhythms. This is a much better way of living for our hearts, instead of inside a chaotic and stressed-filled existence where we live by the seat of our pants. We may struggle to adapt to a daily routine at first, but as soon as we start feeling that powerful, natural rhythm over erratic, dysfunctional ways, we will find much relief and feel so much healthier physiologically, mentally, and physically.

POWER IN THE PRESENT

As time goes by, you'll continue to be amazed by the power of living in the present moment. I have mentioned this a few times before this chapter. Living in the present moment is a milestone in your healing journey, an awakening for those who struggle with anxieties. Once you start to experience the beauty and peace from this, you will embrace it all the time. As you continue to conquer this approach to life, many of your worries, fears and anxieties will disappear. What a fabulous phenomenon!

Why does this correlation exist? Because many of your fears stem from feeling out of control. When you project your thoughts and minds to the future, you can't control it because it is the future. You can only control the current moment. The more fully you live in the present, the more control you will feel. The reverse is also true. If you continually focus or obsess over the past, you will feel possible depressions and less in control because it is the past. Way too much thinking about the future has a tendency to bring on feelings of being overwhelmed, because you cannot control either the past or the illusion of the futures. You will only feel centered and balanced when living in the present moment where you can experience the spontaneous gifts life has to offer.

MOVE THE ENERGY

Feeling good, balanced and optimistic through your first year is also about moving your energy. Stress energies get stuck, in your tissues, your organs, your mind, your heart, and unknowingly becomes stored throughout your whole body. This becomes toxic and you won't feel your best. Understanding that you must move the stressful, toxic energies out of your inner body and replace them with peaceful, healing energies is critical to your heart health. You may not always remember that with every negative thought, action, or experience, negative energy builds up inside. You may not realize that how you sit all day long or even drive in your vehicle builds up toxins inside your body from lack of movement. You must find daily ways in which to remove all this crud from your physical and spiritual bodies that pulls you down and replace it with movement. This will provide you with equanimity where you will feel poised, self-controlled, peaceful, balanced, and calm. What wonderful words!

Something needs to trigger this movement within us, maybe a combination of behaviors. Physical exercise, including yoga and simply walking, can be a great start to relieving the physical stressors and helping us to feel calmer. Any kind of daily exercise for a minimum of thirty minutes needs to become a priority. Stretching, a hot sauna, a hot tub, spinal twists, and other yoga-types of positions can help wring toxins out of our body parts and open room inside for positive energy, rebuilding, and balance. Quiet meditation, if only for five minutes a day, can help move us in the right direction as well and result in level-headedness. The important point is that these activities need to be done consistently, on a daily basis, in order to reach and maintain a physical and mental peace about ourselves. It is all about moving the old, negative, stagnant energies out, while replacing them with healing, positive, and peaceful energies.

We are physical beings that need movement. Once I started to get some type of physical activity in every single day as a result of my cardiac rehab program, I noticed a significant difference in my outlook, feelings, moods, and sleeping habits. I also wasn't tied to a computer for twelve hours a day anymore. We cannot sit all day and night, without movement. We must move our bodies and sweat the toxins out. At the same time, we are spiritual beings that need balancing. Consider starting a routine that includes prayerful meditation, through a yoga practice or time alone at home. You will notice a significant difference in your attitude and feelings, you will be less reactive and this will naturally result in heart health.

NEGATIVE DIALOGUE

Going forward, when you encounter negative talk from the inside or the outside, stay on guard and protect yourself from allowing it to seep into your mind and soul. Negative dialogue is the catalyst for much of people's daily distress, with anxious episodes as the result. Stay away from the "what if" and the "should have" sentences. By doing so, you are protecting your mind, your stomach and gut, and ultimately your heart. Distract yourself with positive action as well as positive mantras. Negative dialogue and self-talk are downers, no matter how you look at it. One thought leads to another and the domino effect takes over. Over time, my physical body pays for this abuse by getting sick from the stress of the anxiety that has resulted. I must take control of the negative thoughts as soon as they creep up. I can start to regain control by asking myself if the thought is real or not. Is the thought based on truth and external facts? If not, then is it internally created? In the above scenario, the first couple of thoughts are reality-based, but the negative thinking spirals into a non-fact-based, non-realistic possibility.

PLANT NEW SEEDS

During this first year, take the time to look around and see that the resources and people in your life that can help you break through any barriers you may have in continuing to plant new seeds in your life. It is so important to continue to grow, learn, and not be stagnant. Do this for your heart because you now know and understand the brain-heart connection. There are people who cross your path that have knowledge, contacts, insights, and compassion to help you plant your seeds and move you forward. It is a responsibility to your heart to identify these individuals: family members, neighbors, clergymen, friends, or work colleagues.

Are there people that you see at the local bookstore all the time, or maybe the family doctor? All you need to do is plant a new seed that starts in your heart, watch it take root and allow it to be nurtured by yourself and others you trust. Be encouraged in knowing that this new seed will grow, new branches will sprout, and fruit will be harvested. I pray that new seeds take root in my heart and grow bountiful harvests in my life. I am filled with hope and expectancy of wonderful things to happen. I just need to stay open to the people, opportunities, and resources that are brought to me every day, and not be blind anymore to the changes that can take place. I healed from my sicknesses and lost the extra pounds. I rid myself of the unhealthy habits and stopped doubting myself. I started believing, once again, that good things and good people are possible.

SAFE AND SOUND

Leaving the fears and frustrations of the world behind us and being home safe and sound is the best feeling in the world for anyone. Many of us may have been blessed, able to spend much of our lives feeling safe and sound in our home, until recently when circumstances have made us doubt our future with energies snuffed out from our health set back or the pandemic. We fully realize that having this safe and sound feeling is a luxury. Concerns and worries that we carry are overwhelming to us, and are taking away our safeness while exhausting us at the same time. Do all that you can to feel and regain that sense of security, love, caring, and safeness in your home again. There's nothing in the world like this comfort.

WRAPPED IN LOVE

There is nothing we can do to protect ourselves from future losses in your life, either from natural causes or painful accidents. When these things happen around you, keep your anxiety and other emotions in check and protect yourself from falling into what I call the "fear-funk." The fear-funk is a period that can last a while and is spurred out of fear. The fear-funk is defined and experienced differently for everyone. For me, I believe my fear is based on the concepts of loss and abandonment, which feeds into my fear-funk core. For you, it very well may be this or other factors. If you fall into a fear-funk, don't be alone. Reach out to your pillar peeps or support network who will help you to bear the pain. If you stay alone, your fear and anxiety may spiral out of control and into panic. Panic is unnerving and upsetting, and feeling out of control results in feeling powerless. Being with others will help you work through this and back to healing.

What I have realized is that when I flip it upside down and reframe the fear-funk concept, I totally see that this emotion is really about me needing to be wrapped in love, at my core, surrounded by people who support me, care for me, love me, and make me feel safe again. Having this epiphany made me want to cry out of joy because I realized that being wrapped in love is only about one thing: healing. Focusing on being wrapped in love, versus being in a fear-funk, is an uplifting and positive dynamic that brings a smile to my face, relief to my heart, mind, body, and soul.

Be careful about interpreting your emotions and feelings that are clouded by fear. Instead, allow yourself to be wrapped in God's love, wrapped in your kids' love, and family love. The plan for me and for you in your first year, post-heart attack, is to stay in a state *wrapped in love* as much as possible. The loving plan is to heal from losses felt from the heart event, from the pandemic, and from losing people in our lives. Continue to pull through life with strength and confidence, powered by grace. There is light, and in that light, this too shall pass and we will be at peace because we are wrapped in love.

SURVIVOR MODE

If you come across difficult and challenging times the first year, and you need some alone time, tell yourself it's okay and move into what I call "survivor mode." This is a phrase used a lot in the house when raising my kids. Whenever the stresses of life got piled too high, with too many unmanaged expectations, I would tell my family that I needed time just for myself because I was operating in "survivor mode." Who knew that one day this would take on a whole new meaning?

I would easily tell friends and family, "Touch base with me in a few days because right now, I am in survivor mode." This sentiment served me well many times and I was able to consciously strip away all the peripheral, non-essential stuff from life and simply concentrate on my most basic priorities and needs. Survivor mode may surface for you when you are enduring a critical life stressor, or a bundle of life stressors. When the going gets tough, strip back to the most basic of needs: taking care of yourself with your healthy habits, and protecting your heart. It becomes so easy now, to redefine our days or activities when we need to because we have our core belief and commitment toward staying healthy. For me, these core healthy things consist of: resting, eating well, walking or other exercise, staying hydrated, conversing with folks and being around those whose energy feeds me, cuddling with my dogs, and engaging only in activities that renew the soul and energy. It's good to mention that hibernation is totally a go-to activity during survivor mode. You will notice when survivor mode starts to fade away because the pressures of life have diminished, relief sets in, and anxieties are at bay. You can then grant yourself permission to rejoin the world.

LIFE IS NOT A MARATHON

It sure feels like life is a marathon sometimes, but is it? Maybe it should be viewed more like a game of chess, adjusting one piece at a time as we move along the continuum of change. Going forward, think of your continued heart journey as a walk along a long, winding river, not running any type of marathon or race. Along this river, learn from the decisions and actions you have already taken. Close your eyes and meditate on these words: take a new path, strategies, methods, and beginnings, optimism, shifting, personalized walking pace, perpetual healing, empowerment, taking control of your future, growth, pressing forward, passing by stagnation, and letting go of the past to make room for your bright future.

Don't the following words sound wonderful, a new beginning, a new start, a stirring within, an arousal? They sound wonderful because they are. They fill you with hope and joy for a better tomorrow. You have already started to address your needed lifestyle changes by making necessary adjustments through the recalibrate step and have taken the steps toward your new beginning. You are awakened and are moving yourself from the early feeling of paralysis to movement and action. You can and will continue to conquer because you are smart, competent, and capable. As you continue to address the lifestyle changes with adjustments as needed, and take action to improve, the load you've been carrying becomes much lighter and eventually disappears. You will find the freedom and peace you deserve and will build the good life you desire.

As you implement the changes in your life that are needed, you will become more motivated to continue and more reassured that the brokenness you have been experiencing will disappear forever. Changing your life forever will be a huge accomplishment and it will allow you to live the life that you so deserve. With this new start and beginning in your life, you will receive hope for positive improvements. The growth will stretch you into newness, brightness, and energy-filled experiences. You will not go back to being unhealthy. Instead, you are in a state of becoming a much better, improved person that can confidently manage your life and heart concerns instead of allowing them to manage you.

OBSTACLES

Being aware of potential obstacles, especially during the first-year post-heart attack, will prevent you from being shocked, scared, thrown off-guard or spiraled into panic when they arise. Instead, you can be prepared to manage them in healthy, non-reactive manners, which will allow you to return to your healthy lifestyle, staying heart-centered. Let's unpack some of the potential, common obstacles: toxic people, monster mind, yearning for the old, procrastination, triggers, hyperarousal, off-balance, eustress, and having a broken heart.

Toxic people will continue to get in your way and impede your healing and new, healthy lifestyle. Because of your struggle, its unpleasantness as well as the growth, you have changed. Your attitudes toward things in life along with your behaviors have all been upgraded. Your view on the world around you and toward your daily life is different. You no longer are the person you were pre-heart attack, and for this, others in your life may or may not continue to embrace you. That's OK. You are strong, courageous, and more than enough, and if space is created by others dropping by the wayside, so be it. This is only a sign that new, beautiful humans will be entering into your life, ones who will bring love, joy, comfort and growth and will support you in your new life and lifestyle ways. Be thankful and let go of the pain that accompanies saying goodbye to those who don't embrace you any longer. It is sad, indeed, but you know all too well that putting energy and effort into trying to make a person want to spend time with you or share their love with you is pointless. You do not deserve this pain. Have enough self-respect to let them go.

Monster Mind

Monsters in your mind will try to distract you from your missions and goals. They will pop up randomly or because of a trigger. Monster mind is when you start to be Negative Nelly and Pessimistic Peter about just about everything. It lurks in the background, waiting to strike when you are feeling down and out and tired. It will try to grab your mind and make you think obsessively about how shitty everything has suddenly become. Specific examples include repetitive negative thought patterns, worrying about future events (waiting for medical test results or job restructuring), or unrealistic, perfectionist expectations. The best thing to do to alleviate this is to get active. When you are active, you are distracted and productive, which takes the monster's power away. Go get some exercise and combat them with producing the feel-good chemicals and hormones that fight monster mind. Grab a friend and chunk out reading this book together and talk strategy. Face your monster thoughts head-on, research them if it is a bothersome topic because knowledge is your power. Kick the monsters to the curb.

Yearning for the Old

There is a sensitive trap that you can fall into during times when you are feeling lonely, vulnerable, and fragile due to the chaos from the world. You may find yourself saying inside your monkey mind, "If only I could be normal again and have things go back to how they were." Even worse than this is if others have casually said to you, "I wish things were back to normal for you." If this starts to happen, it's time to take a step back and re-evaluate. First and foremost, there were so many factors that allowed you the grace to *survive* your heart attack. By saying these types of things or hearing them from others, you are throwing caution to the wind, which literally means to "utterly vanish" or "become out of existence." Thank God that wasn't the case.

Secondly, not honoring the progress you have made in recovery and healing is extremely disrespectful to yourself. You have become a much better, healthier person in so many ways because of the hard physical and mental work you have done: learning all about your heart; embracing new disciplines; using technology; creative thinking;

adapting quickly to change; shifting your thoughts; and so on. Please make your own list in your journal of all that you have learned and benefited from since your heart attack. Make a list of all the ways you have changed because of the pain you have had to endure and how these changes have benefited you.

And, lastly, by saying or thinking that you wish things were back to how they use to be, you risk pulling yourself into denial and feeling like you failed, a state you already faced head on and wiped away. You know in your heart that you're are not a failure, but maybe you are feeling susceptible for some reason at this time. There is probably something else that is going on. Simply cut yourself some slack. Embrace a mantra inside your head or in your journal to push this way. Create your own or repeat this simple logic: My heart has changed, so I have changed and my life has changed. It's all good. It's impossible to be the same person you use to be. Think of it this way: you will always be the sum of every person you have been throughout your life. With that eye-opening thought, how can you possibly be the same? You are a dynamic person in a dynamic world: #fact.

Procrastination

That little beast that may try to eat away at you, tiny bits at a time, savoring every bite, is called "procrastination." You cannot help it. It's just there, existing by our side with that little voice in our heads that tells us to go ahead and move forward. You need to get the job done but can't because you are in a state of procrastination. What do you do? The normal response would be, force yourself do to the X, Y, Z task or thing. Push yourself through it. But we know that doesn't work anymore for us. There is a reason why we are procrastinating, and we have to get to the bottom of this root cause, peel that back and then create a new plan, one that works for you. Your intuitive self is much more engaged and operating at a deeper level now compared to before your heart attack. Respect this. When you have things figured out and are comfortable, you will embrace your inner warrior, take the necessary leap, and go well beyond the comfort zone. It is from a lack of motivating factors that procrastination is created. Answer "why" and you will know what to do. Read the following and embrace it:

I need to accept myself and love myself for who I am. If I am being honest about it, I have yet to take this critical step of truly accepting myself despite what I label as my shortcomings. In doing so, I will give myself the power to push past my fears and anxieties and not let them prevent me from accomplishing the things I want to in my life. I will accept them, feeling them when they happen, having faith that they will not last forever and trust that I can move beyond them. The more I survive these episodes pushing past them, the more successful I will feel.

Triggers

There were a few situations that were triggers for my panic and fear when I first returned home from the hospital. One was the chair I was sitting in when my heart attack first started and the other was the smell of my favorite cup of coffee, the one I was sipping while in the chair when my heart attack came on. It was difficult for me to be home alone with my dog at first. Over time, as I gained different memories while in that chair, I became desensitized and was comfortable in it again. The coffee, not so much. I will have it on occasion but for some reason it still spooks me, and that's OK. There are plenty of other coffees to be enjoying. I am sure there are triggers for you as well, regarding where you were, who you were with, and maybe even smells, like my coffee. Some you will become desensitized to and others possibly not.

My first day at cardiac rehab, they hooked me up to the heart monitor and it threw me for a loop because I hadn't had all those wires on me with the stickers and such since the hospital. I had to breathe through it until I calmed down. After a few sessions and becoming desensitized to it, I was able to hook myself up with the heart monitor with no worries at all.

I also went through a spell where I felt this way about online content, streaming, and other media. Triggers were easily sparked due to hyperarousal. Hyperarousal is a feeling that comes from enduring a time in your life where you underwent a lot of stress. It is a state in which our nervous systems are very sensitive and highly reactive, more so than the normal person. We feel panic and fear as a reaction to situations that we know others do not. We also can have drastic emotional and physical symptoms that others do not when we are in a state of hyperarousal and can be misunderstood by others who are around us in times of hyperarousal. It can be scary, frustrating, and confusing, but at least now we have the right word to put to it! Simply put, we are emotionally and physically vulnerable, fragile, and sensitive, and need to respect this and stay heart focused.

Eustress & Distress

Stress can become an obstacle for you from moving through and completing the steps in this book. But remember, there is a difference between good and bad stress, and you want to be focused on eustress. Eustress is the term for positive stress. An example of eustress is having to complete a PowerPoint for work that is not that challenging to you, or going for a long run. Both are beneficial, can be motivating, use focused energy, and are focused on the positive. If, however, you are asked to present the PowerPoint to a large group of people and you hate doing this type of thing, then that is distress because it is a negative form of stress. In daily life, we often use the term "stress" to describe negative situations. Other forms of distress include divorce, suicide, a car accident, or a life-threatening illness or heart attack. If you have stress in your life which prevents you from working the program in this book, the best thing to do is balance it with eustress experiences, like reading and working the program in this book! Below are some other examples of activities that relieve distress:

- Acupressure, massage, reflexology, or reiki
- Tai Chi, yoga, Shiatsu, or other forms of physical techniques
- Cuddling, kissing, and having sex
- Listening to music
- Chiropractic methods
- Exercise, activity, walking, Pilates, or other forms of movement
- Being in Nature or doing what brings you joy

A Broken Heart

As we discussed earlier, recovering from a broken heart is one of the most painful experiences we can have as human beings and if this happens the first year, it can become an obstacle to your continued healing. It strips us of hope, joy, trust, and all our energy, including the reserves. The suffering, loneliness, and possible feelings of rejection are serious emotional blows to contend with. When an intimate, deep relationship we have is fractured, lost, or broken, the distress and loss weigh heavily on our hearts. We need to be very careful to prevent further heart damage or another event from occurring during this time of grieving. Your mindful goal at a time like this is to one hundred protect yourself and your heart, and not to slip into a state of negligence. Work through your grief and have a speedy recovery from the loss that moves you to regain a positive outlook. You hand-picked your pillar people, created your family and friend network, and have medical staff for support. It is time to lean on them and not tackle this alone. Seek out medical attention at any time as well as counseling or therapy. Do not discontinue your medications, isolate, or withdraw from your life. You have come too far and have the strength you need to face this set-back. Have your friends and family help you stick to your regime.

Off-Balance

There will be times when you simply feel off-balance and don't have the gusto for finishing the steps, doing the work, or reading. That's OK. It just means other stuff is going on in your life. But, soon enough, you will hopefully carve out the time to re-center yourself, and perhaps say no to something else in order to focus on this book. Saying "no" to others is okay, especially if you are way overbooked with a slammed schedule. If it is a case of being too passive and having difficulty saying no, practice it by being assertive politely, not aggressively, and with respect to others. Remember to politely decline requests made of you that are not heart-healthy. Yes, it is hard, but remember any harm to your heart takes away from advancing your mission. Consider that not being able to say no can bring on a considerable amount of stress by your becoming overwhelmed. Taking fifteen minutes of your day to dedicate efforts to this book and you will receive the value, the benefits for the quality of your life.

14

MAY YOUR HEART SOAR

"Never give up. No matter what is going on. Never give up. Develop the heart. Too much energy in your country is spent on developing the mind instead of the heart ... work for peace in your heart and in the world. Work for peace and I say again: Never give up. No matter what is going on around you. Never give up."

— THE DALAI LAMA

Congratulations on reading through this book, working the steps of the Heart Healing Process, and getting to the last chapter. There were so many unknown and grey areas at the start of your process that are now turned around. At the beginning of the book, I promised to lay out the roadmap to help you through recovery and healing. To do that, you needed to work through the steps to understand your condition(s), how your heart attack happened, why it happened, and what needs changing to prevent another one. This roadmap, in conjunction with working with your cardiologist and your medical program, provides you with the tools needed to move past your fear, regain your confidence, and restore control. The roadmap is a process to guide you through recovery and healing but also something you can refer to in times of need or setback.

If, by chance, you have not read this book and skipped to the last chapter, I will need to tell you that what is covered in this chapter alone will not help you move past your post-heart attack fear. In order to achieve this, there is a full process that one needs to go through during recovery and healing in order to receive the valuable benefits, including letting go of fear.

By dedicating precious time to reading this book, you were able to acquire the knowledge needed to answer the question, "why did I have a heart attack?" and to face your conditions head on. You've discovered a lot around mental mastery and its vital connection to the full healing and recovery process. With the wrong, negative mindset, healing is not possible. With a healthy, supported positive mindset, nothing is impossible. You have learned the critical importance around having a loving, winning community of support as you travel through the stages of grief. It is very difficult to recover and heal, mentally and physically, if you are surrounded by people who do not understand what you experienced and what you are enduring. Through your cardiac rehab, medical staff, and other heart attack victim stories, you have received the help and guidance you need. Your strong, new healthy lifestyle is your new foundation for life. Through the power of good habits and routine, you can maintain your new, powerful ways of living.

MINDSET TO HEART-SET

Every heart journey is different because every heart attack survivor brings their own story to life with their own unique nuances and needs for recovery and healing. However, there is one thing common amongst all victims and that is fear. We suffer from fear of having another heart attack, from not fully recovering, not being able to live your best life, from rejection, judgment, and future discrimination. We suffer from the fear that the damage to our hearts will not heal. Basically, there is a shit-ton of fear. But the radical difference with you is that you have had the courage to take the bull by the horns, make the commitment to yourself to take the time to face recovery and healing, and now you are creating a new, healthy life. Be ignited with confidence because that makes all the difference! Fear was oozing all over the place when you started this book/ heart journey, now it just drip… drip… drips… a tiny bit here and there. Writing and sharing this book about the path that worked for me to benefit others has been my difference and helped pushed me past the fears. Having a heart attack also, in and of itself, helps a survivor throw fear to the curb because we are survivors.

TRANSFORMATION TRAITS

Your physical energies allow you to focus on tasks at hand with a love-filled heart for your family and friends. You can continue to have peace and joy all through your body with a clear mind because every day you can scrape away the crap that tries to push and hold you down. Obsessions and anxious thoughts are not recipients of any of your attention, and you are finding simple joy and gratitude throughout your daily activities and chores.

Don't be surprised if you have weepy days like I did and still do, where you cry out of nowhere, but you know it's from the overwhelming feeling of relief and gratitude for still being able to experience this world. You have just traveled through a long, dark hallway that was scary and surrounded you with doubt, fear, and concern. You held on tight, maybe too tight at times, but you pulled out all the tools you had and found the strength to crack open some windows and doors to let the light in. Maybe you turned it over to your God, Source, or Higher Power to hold you in loving arms as you traversed through that dark hall. Maybe you reached out to your guardian angels who helped you through recovery and healing. You are here, now, and you have your heart to thank for it. It stayed strong for you, hanging on in its damaged and fragile capacity when you needed it the most.

Today is a wonderful day to be living, as is any day, truth be told. It is through discovering your Truth that you can start living freely. Mysteries solved, hidden discoveries of strength made, and all the work you've completed within these chapters create a new start. You will go forward in life, free from fear and embracing the goodness in your healthy life, full of well-being. Let your light shine bright on the inside and outside and know that feeling good is possible and amazing. You deserve this. You will have many more days, weeks, months, and years like this because you know how to keep your spirits on the path of healing, goodness, light, and health.

ZEST FOR LIFE

With your healthy lifestyle in place, you will move through life with confidence, joy, and a deep zest for living! The negative patterns of thinking, doing, and being are tamed now, and you control your life with positivity and knowing how to surround yourself with energy that feeds your soul. Now is the time to make plans for your future! Where do you want to go? Who do you want to see? What kind of experiences do you want to have? When you are involved with making plans, the front part of your brain known as the prefrontal cortex, is activated in order to accomplish this process. As a result, dopamine is released, a chemical that elevates your mood in good ways. Having positive emotions stimulated is excellent for you and helps to battle any stress. Plan to go visit friends, family, or new places that you have always wanted to visit. Even planning to go to the local farmers market on Saturdays with friends is excellent for your brain and, now you also know, for your heart. You will be so much less tense, and more energetic while doing all the things you love again.

BE THE BEST VERSION OF YOU

You have successfully manifested an amazing new version of yourself. You are different because of your life changing experience, and you are very special because you survived it. As a result of this miraculous event, the love you have for your heart has increased ten-fold and the respect you hold for its magnificence is off the charts. As a result of applying the methods in this book, you have learned the real Truth about your circumstance and have gotten in touch with the real reasons for why it happened. Many people who don't take the time to be their best detective stay lost, have difficulties connecting to the world again, and have challenges figuring out their new normal post-heart event. You have done the work and unclogged your mental system, tackled the kaleidoscope of emotions, and worked through the process to uncover all the layers that were getting in the way of your healing.

I say to you, continue breaking out of your cocoon, embrace life with gusto, and keep on deeply loving. Let go of any leftover internal conflict because you know what's needed to move on. There is no reason whatsoever to beat yourself up any more about anything, because you know what changes need to be made to keep your protective shield up. Your demons have been uncovered and buried. You've worked hard on the process and this sets you free. Most of all, forgive yourself and say a final goodbye to any guilt that follows you around. You deserve nothing but inner peace, with a calm heart, within the constructed walls you've built around your life.

BEYOND BLESSED

Your heart attack came at a time when you couldn't be more blessed. You may be asking yourself, how in the hell was it a blessed time? Because it happened after there has been tremendous advances in the practice of cardiology, health care, and rehab therapy. Prior to this day and age, you may very well have faced a much graver outcome, or one of a severely confined existence. Modern medicine's progress has been phenomenal and as a result, you have been the recipient of life saving procedures, therapeutic methods, and medical management practices that allowed you to survive to go on to live an abundant life. Now go live it!

APPENDIX: HEALTHY HEART NUTRITION

By Courtney Steele George, MPH in Nutrition, University of North Carolina, Chapel Hill

SECTION 1: HEART HEALTHY FOOD AND LIFESTYLE MANTRAS

Below are phrases to be repeated in a meditative way, in a concentrated manner, that will help instill new ways of thinking, believing and behaving.

- I will make slow, life-long lifestyle nutrition and diet changes to improve my health and happiness, not just short-term dieting and repressing myself in the short-term.
- I will be consistently working with my healthcare team, which can include a cardiologist, primary care provider, dietitian, physical therapist, psychiatrist, life coach, fitness instructor, et cetera, who can help me achieve my long-term lifestyle goals.

- I will use food, nutrition, and exercise as my first-line medicine, along with other medical treatments recommended to me by my healthcare providers.
- I will continue to take care of my mental, spiritual, and emotional wellness, which affects all other parts of my health, including my heart.
- I will do my very best to implement recommendations of a heart healthy diet and dietary guidelines for Americans (see below), which includes emphasizing produce, legumes, nuts, fish, and lots of exercise.
- I will continue to monitor indicators which are concerning for my health condition, such as sodium intake, adequate hydration, blood pressure, breathing, stress, et cetera, and be mindful of these factors on my overall health.
- I will continue to love myself and my body over everything else, and will prioritize the importance of my health and happiness. My body is an amazing machine, which wants me to heal and be healthy.

SECTION 2: NUTRITION RECOMMENDATIONS AND SOURCES

Below are resources for you to check out in detail on recommended heart healthy dietary patterns.

Source 1: American Dietary Guidelines - https://www.dietaryguidelines.gov/

> These are the general healthy eating guidelines revised every five years by the top nutrition experts

around the country and then reviewed by the USDA and DHHS. Their online tool allows you to customize to fit your needs.

Source 2: AHA - https://www.heart.org/en/healthy-living/healthy-eating

This is the leading research organization on heart health, other than the NIH, and they have a whole landing page full of nutrition and healthy living tips.

Source 3: DASH Diet - https://www.nhlbi.nih.gov/health-topics/dash-eating-plan

This is the NIH website information page on the well-researched DASH diet, known as the Dietary Approaches to Stop Hypertension.

Source 4: Mediterranean Diet

There isn't one source which defines exactly what the Mediterranean diet entails, so I have included many different sources here. They all share similar themes, like high quantities of fruits and vegetables, fish, olive oil, and exercise.

- https://www.heart.org/en/healthy-living/healthy-eating/eat-smart/nutrition-basics/mediterranean-diet
- https://www.webmd.com/diet/a-z/the-mediterranean-diet
- https://www.mayoclinic.org/healthy-lifestyle/nutrition-and-healthy-eating/in-depth/mediterranean-diet/art-20047801

- https://pubmed.ncbi.nlm.nih.gov/25447615/

SECTION 3: HEART HEALTHY PANTRY IDEAS

Here is a list of items to keep on hand in the pantry at all times, to help you in making easy, heart-healthy recipes.

- Canned tomatoes, tomato sauce, and paste: perfect for impromptu dishes like pasta, vegetables, curry, or can be added to any soups. Make sure to look for lower sodium versions. Remember too that adding greens to any dish greatly increases your nutrition and fiber. Spinach, for example, can always be added to dishes, sandwiches, omelets, et cetera.
- Favorite canned vegetables: Corn, green beans, peas, beets, mixed vegetables.
- Favorite dried beans and pulses: Lentils, black-eyed peas, pinto beans, kidney beans, whatever you like to eat. You can even have some cans on hand as well, but again, those tend to be high in sodium.
- Favorite spices: You want to stock up on different spices and herbs to utilize so that you can flavor your dishes without having to add as much sugar, sodium, and fats to meals. Some of my favorites are Italian seasoning, pumpkin spice seasoning, cumin, and fresh ground pepper. This can also become something new for you to try: learning how to use new spices.
- Frozen fruits and vegetables: Again, this should be anything that you would use a lot, especially for making morning protein shakes. Adding a frozen fruit to the blender is a great way to add

flavor and nutrition. You never want to run out of having access to produce, so don't let a run to the store get in your way of getting your fruits and veggies in! Having them in the freezer is wildly convenient and great for soups, stir-fry, and smoothies.
- Nutritional yeast: This is a low-sodium, dairy-free option for people who still want a savory topping for everything that you would put parmesan cheese on, like salads, popcorn, soups, et cetera.
- Canned fish: Many fish have heart healthy omega-3 fatty acids and in general are good protein sources, compared to other animal foods, for cardiovascular disease.

SECTION 4: INTUITIVE EATING

The modern-day nutrition concept of "Intuitive Eating" was developed by two dietitians, but the basic tenants have been around for a long time. The biggest takeaway from intuitive eating is that it puts your body back into the driver's seat for your food decisions, rather than diet culture, shame, or emotional eating. According to the experts, if you follow these ten principles as much as possible, you will live a happier, healthier, more mindful life, while being less at-odds with your body. This was taken extensively from: https://www.intuitiveeating.org/10-principles-of-intuitive-eating/

1. Reject the "Diet" Mentality

Basically, diets will not help you, but instead hurt the connection you have with your body's hunger/ satiety cues. The journey of intuitive eating starts here.

2. Honor Your Hunger

Hunger is a natural feeling sent by the brain to the gut to stimulate you to eat, and sometimes even to eat specific foods as well. This is the first crucial step to eating based on your intuition and body signals, instead of by a diet.

3. Make Peace with Food

Nutritious, whole food is not the enemy, it is your friend because it gives you the nutrients and energy you need to live your life – like going to the store, working, playing with your dog outside, and exercising. Another crucial step in intuitive eating is to reject the morality put on some foods and not others, and reject the idea that food and your hunger are the enemies to your health goals.

4. Challenge the Food Police

Reject people, media, and thoughts which try to police your food choices and hunger feelings. You are the only one who knows your body and your body knows your cues, plus you have been educated now on nutritious eating habits with heart healthy wholeness.

5. Discover the Satisfaction Factor

Go on an eating journey with yourself to discover what really satisfies your hunger cues, what keeps you satiated, and what works for you, based on this new mindfulness with your body guiding you.

6. Feel Your Fullness

When you feel full, respect it. It is not good or bad. It's simply a message sent from your gut to your brain telling you that you have eaten enough. Sometimes you will want to feel full and sometimes you will feel less interested in eating a lot – that is the natural ebb and flow of the body. This also means respecting this fullness and not eating anymore. If you are eating while full, then these next principles are for you.

7. Cope with Your Emotions with Kindness

According to the *10 Principles on Intuitive Eating*, this is crucial. "First, recognize that food restriction, both physically and mentally, can, in and of itself, trigger loss of control, which can feel like emotional eating. Find kind ways to comfort, nurture, distract, and resolve your issues. Anxiety, loneliness, boredom, and anger are emotions we all experience throughout life. Each has its own trigger, and each has its own appeasement. Food won't fix any of these feelings. It may comfort for the short term, distract from the pain, or even numb you. But food won't solve the problem. If anything, eating for an emotional hunger may only make you feel worse in the long run. You'll ultimately have to deal with the source of the emotion."

8. Respect Your Body

"Accept your genetic blueprint. Just as a person with a shoe size of eight would not expect to realistically squeeze into a size six, it is equally futile (and uncomfortable) to have a similar expectation about body size. But mostly, respect your body so you can feel better about who you are. It's hard to reject the diet mentality if you are unrealistic and overly critical of your body size or shape. All bodies deserve dignity."

If you have further interest in this principle, please check out the Health at Every Size movement happening in the healthcare industry and on social media.

9. Movement—Feel the Difference

The intuitive eating developers want to expand the principles in this to exercise as well. The same ideas apply: listen to your body, don't overdo it and hurt yourself, love the body which allows you to exercise, and don't use it as punishment, but as enjoyment. Find something you enjoy doing, and it will benefit you physically and mentally.

10. Honor Your Health—Gentle Nutrition

Another way of stating this last principle is something which is very popular now among many dietitians, which is the 80/20 rule. This means that around 80 percent, or the majority, of your nutrition and lifestyle choices should be with your health and intuitive eating in mind. The other 20 percent is for pleasure, holidays, traditions, whatever you would like.

SECTION 5: EXAMPLES OF EVIDENCE-BASED RESOURCES TO FURTHER ANSWER YOUR NUTRITION QUESTIONS

No study, book, or even set of recommendations can be exhaustive of all the information there is on nutrition that you might want to know about. It is only natural that you might have further questions beyond this appendix, so here are some basic tips on how to get credible information you need to make evidence-based health decisions for your future.

- If you can, seek nutritional counsel. Usually your local hospital will have a dietitian on staff to help you make more heart healthy choices, so check there first. While this isn't possible for everyone, since dietitian counseling is not always covered by all insurance, just one consulting over Telehealth could be very helpful in answering your questions and getting you on the right path to achieving heart health. Dietitians are also the only licensed professionals with the proper training to give nutrition advice for heart attack survivors.
- If you can't go with Option One, then there is a wealth of nutrition resources out there. I will list some here, but what you want to look for is information based on recommendations and

studies told by trained professionals. Even if a book or blog is written by someone with a degree, if it isn't a Registered Dietitian Degree, then I encourage you to remain skeptical.
- Some good online resources to consider are listed here:

1. www.eatright.org is the website of the Academy of Nutrition and Dietetics

2. https://pubmed.ncbi.nlm.nih.gov/ is the official scientific search engine from the National Library of Medicine to find health information and recent journal publications

ACKNOWLEDGMENTS

To my precious children, Courtney and Dalton, for pushing me beyond the walls of living a blueprint life. For blooming into their amazing, authentic selves. For teaching me how to embrace and live my authentic life as well. For dedicating their life work to the improvements of society, the climate, food source, safety, and security, the healthy well-being of others and for their reverence for science. For being among God's gifts, that are blessings to the world, who continue to give throughout their lives. Stay heart-centered and leading life with Love.

Thank you to Geri Brown, A.K.A. Ger-Bear, for being my BFF-sister these last thirty years. For peddling that bike when I've been in the basket, sharing your amazing craziness, always believing in me, having my back, and for fighting our inner gremlins together! We have so much more life to go: Plan A, B, or C!

Many hugs and much love to David for helping with Nahla-dog's care, especially when I needed full rest, for doing all the yard work, keeping the lawn looking good, making the best buffalo nachos and vodka tonics (tall with two limes), and remaining a most wonderful father.

Gratitude to my beautiful sister Cindy for her support, especially for watching over me while we were growing up and taking such loving care of me during my childhood. May life unfold in kind ways for you and all your loved ones, bringing more lovely rainbows on your journey.

Finally, to heart attack survivors everywhere. You are amazing, precious and courageous human beings who have survived that which many do not! Take your newfound strength and fill your hearts with Love. Go forward knowing that the best is yet to come.

ABOUT THE AUTHOR

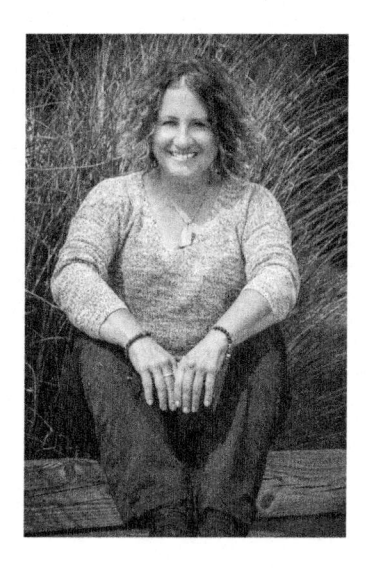

Lisa Steele George MA, RYT, is the founder and CEO of My Heart is Free Life Coaching practice and author of her second book, *Break Free from Heart Attack Fear: The Survivor's Guide to Embrace Your Truth, Regain Confidence & Restore Control.*

A heart attack survivor herself, Lisa supports others with their survivorship and strongly promotes taking the proper time to recover emotionally and physically from a heart event for the deepest healing to occur. Lisa's Heart Healing Process helps survivors transition into living their most vibrant life.

Lisa has two undergrad degrees from University of

Michigan and a master's degree from Michigan State University. As a certified Whole Healing Life (WLH) Coach, accredited by the American Association of Natural Wellness Practitioners (AANWP), Lisa continues mentoring students of Whole Life Healing Center as part of the WLH Collective and enjoys leveraging her thirty-year corporate executive skills in her coaching practice.

As a certified yoga instructor, Lisa enjoys teaching kids' yoga and restorative Yin the most. She is a mother of two adult kids and lives in Rochester Hills, Michigan. Lisa grew up in Clarkston, Michigan but spent most of her summers at Interlochen, where she dedicated herself to her first love, the piano. Rescuing dogs, reading, journaling, travel, water sports, Jeep adventures, and collecting cool coffee mugs are some of Lisa's joys. She can be reached via email at Lisa@Myheartisfree.com.

Website: myheartisfree.com
Facebook: https://www.facebook.com/hearthealingprocess

ABOUT DIFFERENCE PRESS

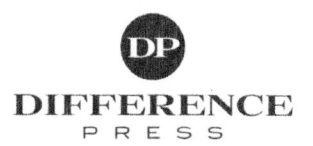

DIFFERENCE
P R E S S

Difference Press is the exclusive publishing arm of The Author Incubator, an educational company for entrepreneurs – including life coaches, healers, consultants, and community leaders – looking for a comprehensive solution to get their books written, published, and promoted. Its founder, Dr. Angela Lauria, has been bringing to life the literary ventures of hundreds of authors-in-transformation since 1994.

A boutique-style self-publishing service for clients of The Author Incubator, Difference Press boasts a fair and easy-to-understand profit structure, low-priced author copies, and author-friendly contract terms. Most importantly, all of our #incubatedauthors maintain ownership of their copyright at all times.

LET'S START A MOVEMENT WITH YOUR MESSAGE

In a market where hundreds of thousands of books are published every year and are never heard from again, The

Author Incubator is different. Not only do all Difference Press books reach Amazon bestseller status, but all of our authors are actively changing lives and making a difference.

Since launching in 2013, we've served over 500 authors who came to us with an idea for a book and were able to write it and get it self-published in less than 6 months. In addition, more than 100 of those books were picked up by traditional publishers and are now available in bookstores. We do this by selecting the highest quality and highest potential applicants for our future programs.

Our program doesn't only teach you how to write a book – our team of coaches, developmental editors, copy editors, art directors, and marketing experts incubate you from having a book idea to being a published, bestselling author, ensuring that the book you create can actually make a difference in the world. Then we give you the training you need to use your book to make the difference in the world, or to create a business out of serving your readers.

ARE YOU READY TO MAKE A DIFFERENCE?

You've seen other people make a difference with a book. Now it's your turn. If you are ready to stop watching and start taking massive action, go to http://theauthorincubator.com/apply/.

"Yes, I'm ready!"

OTHER BOOKS BY DIFFERENCE PRESS

Start Thriving as a Coach!: Release Your Money Blocks and Learn to Manifest Like a Master by Betty Barnett

The Gutsy Wife's Guide to Save Your Marriage: Six Steps to Master Effective Communication with Your Husband by Kimberly H. Brenner

Ultimate Connection: The Blueprint to Everlasting Love Inside Yourself by Dr. Carolyn DeLucia

Making Spirt-Led Decisions for Your Marriage: Unlock the Right Answer for Your Relationship by Ginny Ellsworth

Your Body is Your Superpower: How to Live with Confidence, Courage, and Joy by Janet Farnsworth, MSW

Alchemize Your Divorce: Turn the Toxic Stress of Your Marriage into Abundant Energy for Life by Dr. Kimberly Glow

Freedom from Stress, the Horse's Way: How Equine Facilitated Coaching Can Help You Heal and Thrive by Anna Harold

You Can Have Both: The Guilt-Proof Guide to Managing Your Relationship like You Do Your Business by Chenire Harrell-Carter

Dynamic Equity: Lead Your Team Successfully through Extraordinary Racial Change by Dr. Stephen McCray

Authentic Leadership: The Guide to Be a Spiritual Leader in Your Community by Kristin Panek

Rest, Listen, Love: Learn to Live Joyfully with Chronic Pain by Kendra Sandoval

To Change or Not to Change: 8 Steps to Get Comfortable with Taking Risks and Making Big Life Decisions by Karina Ferrar

I'm Not Jealous: The Ethical Non-Monogamist's Guide to Free Love Relationships without Suffering by S. Sequoia Stafford

Rehabbing the Last 10%: Solutions for Patients Who Have Plateaued during Physical Therapy by Dr. Jennifer Stebbing, DO

The Art of Getting Unstuck: The African American Man's Journey from Surviving to Thriving by Arraina Thomas

The Accidental Alpha Woman: The Guide to Thriving When Life Feels Overwhelming by Karen Wright

THANK YOU

Thank you, readers, from the bottom of my healthy heart, for opening and reading this book. I honor you for your commitment and trust in the content, in yourself and in working through its secret sauce: The Heart Healing Process. It means the world to me that you have as much knowledge as possible to enable your recovery, healing, and long-term well-being. The pages within this book originated from deep within my heart and soul and are lovingly shared to support you. Congratulations on having the courage to take yourself to the next level and unleashing the growth from within!

Since you've finished reading this book, I know you are on the path to regaining your confidence and restoring control. I am so proud of your courage, faith, and trust in yourself. The ground beneath you collapsed and your world shook to the core. But somehow, this book made its way into your life to help get you unstuck and move you forward. I hope that your experience in reading this book is as magical and fulfilling as it was for me while writing it.

Uncovering your Heart-Truth is paramount to your ability to speak and live your Truth. Stay one hundred percent dedicated to leading your life heart-first, while following through with your calls to action. Continue creating that which you need and want in your new post-event world. You deserve all that your heart desires because you have courageously risen from wounded ways.

As a thank you, I've created a meditation series based upon the Heart Healing Process steps that will give you even more motivation, support, and encouragement through your recovery and healing. Please go to the website and sign up to receive them at www.myheartisfree.com. Grab your favorite beverage and sink into a meditation for a few minutes each day. I remain passionate about helping heart attack victims with their recovery and healing process, so please keep in touch and feel free to reach out to me directly about your journey: Lisa@myheartisfree.com. You would be amazed at how many people's lives have been touched by a heart event, and I cherish enriched conversations about the topic.

Most importantly, please make a commitment to share this book with those you know that may have had a heart event, those you love who have a family history of heart problems, and definitely share this book with *all* female friends and family members. Increasing awareness that heart disease is the number one leading cause of death for women is vital in prevention. Don't let your journey end here. Press on to share with others what you have learned and educate them so that you can help save someone else's life, literally.

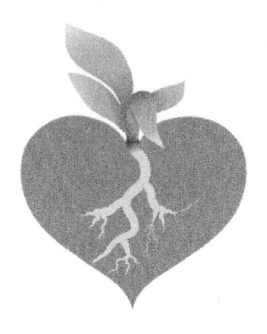

www.myheartisfree.com

Printed in Great Britain
by Amazon